Brain Dance

My Journey with Invisible Illness, Second Chances, and the Wonders of Applied Neuroscience

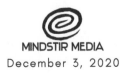

Diane Grimard Wilson

MINDSTIR MEDIA

December 3, 2020

Published by Mindstir Media, LLC
45 Lafayette Rd | Suite 181| North Hampton, NH 03862 | USA
1.800.767.0531 | www.mindstirmedia.com

Printed in the United States of America

ISBN-13: 978-1-7365224-3-1

"I love *Brain Dance*. Diane Wilson is a gifted writer. It read extremely well. I truly got a personal sense of what she went through with her concussions — and all the treatments. Learned plenty I never knew before."

— *Jim Dwyer, MD, Broadcaster (MediBlurb.com),*
Horseman (personal concussion experience)

"*Brain Dance* is a wonderful book. Beautifully written and so needed!"

— *Inna Khazan, PhD, BCB, Clinical Psychologist, Harvard Medical School*

"If you or a loved one has suffered from a concussion or prolonged post-concussive symptoms, *Brain Dance* offers hope and insight. Wilson's experiences as both a patient and a neuroscience professional gives her an authentic and compassionate voice as she gently guides the reader through a vast array of treatment modalities. There are no easy answers or "quick fixes" to brain injuries, but *Brain Dance* shares new resources that address the whole person, including and beyond the conventional options, offering a comprehensive roadmap to recovery."

— *Jill Grimes, MD, FAAFP, Austin, TX,*
Author of The Ultimate College Student Health Handbook

"Diane Wilson has written a compelling account of her struggle with brain trauma in a very readable and intriguing way. Her sense of humor and down-to-earth manner of speaking about what happened and how she followed her gut to heal herself read like a mystery novel I couldn't put down. Bravo!"

— *June Tanoue, MPH, Zen Priest/Teacher,*
Co-Founder Zen Life & Meditation Center, Chicago

"This is a captivating book, once I started reading it I couldn't put it down and finished it in two days. *Brain Dance* is a frank and intimate account of one person's heroic struggle to overcome one of the most commonly undiagnosed health problems in the US today. Diane Wilson explores the various emerging solutions to head trauma, especially neurofeedback, while revealing the many overlooked indicators in our daily life that may be pointing to an unsuspected and very real problem in many of our lives. Diane will help you better understand your symptoms and help you put together your own personal tool kit for traveling the road to recovery."

— *Richard Soutar, PhD, BCN, Founder,*
NewMind Technologies, Author of Doing Neurofeedback: An Introduction

"Diane's story is as important for advancing medicine as the science she shares. She beautifully bridges the gaps in conventional care and turns her injury into an initiation into a new field and skills to help others."

— *Melanie Weller, Medical Visionary, Vagus Nerve Expert*

"This is an extremely powerful and inspiring story that is so applicable right now. It is a solace to those that go through similar experiences and have trouble finding answers to their changes in behavior and emotions. It is so hopeful to hear Diane's story and know that others can relate and feel they are not alone."

— *Maddie Girardi, PT, DPT, CMTPT, Physical Therapist, Chicago*

"Loved the book. I'll recommend it to all of my patients with life-altering health issues."

— *Saul Rosenthal, PhD, BCB, BCB-HRV, BCN, Clinical Health Psychologist*

"I found it hard to set down *Brain Dance* – it was so captivating and written from such a personal and approachable perspective. I can easily see this book becoming an enthralling movie!"

— *Dr. Céleste Grimard, Professor of Leadership, Université du Québec à Montréal, Author of 101 Exercises for Developing Your Leadership*

"With *Brain Dance*, Diane Wilson has written an exceptional book, a must-read for survivors of a brain injury, especially those with post-concussive syndrome, and their loved ones and medical providers. It is important for clinicians to read *Brain Dance* and understand the nuances of the 'invisible injury,' which can present with varying and often life-altering symptoms. As Director of Outpatient Rehabilitation Psychology in one of the top rehabilitation hospitals in the country, I will be strongly recommending this book."

— *Sarah Gray, Psy.D., Clinical Health Psychologist, Instructor, Harvard Medical School and Director of Integrative Psychology, PC*

"For all those with "unseen" illnesses or injuries, this book will show you that you are not alone. Diane Wilson does a masterful job of taking the reader inside the world of someone suffering from a traumatic brain injury."

— *Laura Wimbish-Vanderbeck, Ph.D., Clinical Psychologist, NC*

"I think this is a must read for clinicians, TBI clients and their friends and family. It is a very personal story which will help people understand what you and others go through. But it also includes references to science and science-based therapies that can be very helpful for people who have suffered such an injury."

— *Kathy Abbott, Psy.D., BCN, Clinical Psychologist, Chicago*

"I read Diane's book with great pleasure. Dr. Elsa Baehr is my mother and I had the privilege of working for her for several years designing a brain training program. During this time I met Diane, my mother's neurofeedback intern. Reading *Brain Dance* makes me appreciate Diane and her work even more. This journey to good brain health is an amazing read."

— *Joanne Telser-Frère, DTM, Literacy Chicago*

"*Brain Dance* is a remarkable revelation of a book. Diane invites us along for an engaging, accessible, intimate and memorable journey of diagnosis and recovery — her wit and wonder always intact. *Brain Dance*, ultimately, is not only about the struggle to diagnose and recover from a traumatic brain injury. It is also a guide to nurturing the resilience, perseverance and courage we need to dare to reinvent."

— *Katherine Foran, Editor, Columbia, MO*

"This is a beautiful book! It is both inspiring and a wealth of information. Structured in a framework for brain injury recovery and brain healing that is unique and powerful."

— *Amy Edgar, APRN, CRNP, FNP-C Family Medicine, Allentown, PA*

"Diane Wilson's book is a wonderful resource. She tells her personal experience as a brain injury survivor integrated with her experience as a psychotherapist, coach and neuroscientist. This book is a must read for everyone coping with vehicular trauma and TBI."

— *James F. Zender, PhD, Author Recovering from Your Car Accident:*
The Complete Guide to Reclaiming Your Life.

"Diane's beautiful story gives hope and a roadmap to those suffering traumatic brain injuries. *Brain Dance* is a celebration of possibilities!"

— *Toby Dorr, Author*

"A very well written and compelling story of Diane Wilson's journey with concussion. This book contains a wealth of useful information about the brain and neuroscience, and how it can be used to treat TBI."

— *Roshi Robert Joshin Althouse, Abbot, Zen Life & Meditation Center, Chicago*

" . . . While reading this, I found myself cheering on her recovery and applauding the steps she took to that end, including non-traditional therapies . . . I highly recommend this book for anyone who wants to be inspired to overcome difficulties and set-backs in life."

— *Linda Girgis MD, FAAP, Editor in Chief of Physicians Weekly*

Brain Dance truly will help people. Wilson writes from her heart, using her good head that benefitted from years of diverse treatments, including recruiting neuroplasticity by training her brain with neurofeedback. The world is ready for Wilson's message.

Lynda Thompson, PhD, C.Psych. Distinguished Scientist Award from
AAPB (jointly with Michael Thompson, M.D.)

Contents

Contents

Introduction

As I have trained myself, when my stomach starts getting that sick, acidic feeling and the tension creeps up through my esophagus into the back of my throat, I breathe in deeply, focus on my heart, and then try to gently observe my surroundings. The ballroom of the landmark Fairmont Copley Plaza Hotel in Boston is majestic. The gold-patterned Renaissance-inspired ceiling seems an easy three stories high. Exquisitely detailed, plaster sculpted garlands drape the top of the walls like a wedding cake. As I calm a little, I notice the crystal chandeliers that sprinkle down and dance across the room and grace it with the perfect level of light for focus and comfort. The room is covered with a semi-plush, red diamond pattern carpet, and the air smells slightly like fresh coffee—the expensive kind served not in paper but ceramic cups. The beautiful room is brimming with health care professionals, mainly physicians, for a publishing conference in a style that only the Harvard Medical School could achieve. I'm guessing about that last part, though—whether Harvard Med does it better—since I have never attended a conference at any medical school. Ever.

This situation is a curious first for me. With my counseling degree, I am an MA (Master of Arts) in a sea of MDs (Medical Doctors). The catalyst for this registration was a brochure and mention on Twitter by one of the presenters at this esteemed health care publishing conference, Dr. Linda Girgis. Since I was working on a book, I asked her about it. She asked about my writing. I told her my story, and she encouraged me to attend. Maybe she tells that to everyone, but she seemed sincere and very nice. So, I registered, flew in from Chicago, and showed up. None of that being as easy as it sounds, of course.

Today, this afternoon is the last of the three-day conference. I have been sitting for two hours at a long, linen-covered table in one of the many rows about half-way back from the front, waiting for my number to be called. Kristin, the tall, athletic, sandy blonde woman next to me, has a growing stack of used tissues wadded up in front of her next to an oversized bottle of hand sanitizer. She struggles to manage the waterfall of mucus flowing from her nose. It's her third day of a miserable cold, but we had silently bonded on the first day. During one bad drippy nose moment, I shyly poured her a glass of water from the icy glass pitcher in front of us. She smiled a little. Even in her misery, she knew I had her back. And today, she had mine.

The publishing conference finale involves giving a seventy-second presentation, a pitch on our projects in front of 350 participants, mainly physicians and a group of twenty judges, comprised of literary agents, publishers, book coaches, and retailers. It is led by Dr. Julie Silver, a professor at the Harvard School of Medicine. I had signed up for this pitch portion of the publishing conference along with seventy other brave participants.

I listen as, one by one, impressive people give impressive pitches about their books. There's a president's physician who has worked for more than two administrations in the White House, a neurologist and professor from the Harvard Medical School, deans and other faculty of Ivy League medical schools and other medical schools on both coasts and in the middle of the United States, best-selling authors with sequels to important health books. I wait and wait for my number to be called.

What am I doing here? What was I thinking signing up for this?

Finally, when number 98 is called, I stand up and stride to the front room and stand "on deck" with other presenters who join me in a small group hug. It wasn't only the world's most intense fear—public speaking—kicking in for me. I was describing a book on the most horrible and potentially shaming event of my life.

My name is called, and I stalk across the front of the stage. Not that I felt that confident, I hope that walking hard will grip my high heels into the floor mat and help me not trip. I lock sight on the podium, take the three steps up, adjust the microphone for my tall body, and am given the signal. I am frozen on the inside, my brain... I can feel the attention of the room warm on my face. So many faces out there. A friendly and attentive audience.

"This is a memoir of an invisible illness, one that I could not see myself. Those who knew, no one wanted to talk about with me, that had no cure. That profoundly affected every second of my life."

The moment is far more moving than I had expected, and in the front rows, I see expressions soften, and a woman in the second row dabs her eyes. "It's a story of being a brain injury survivor for whom traditional medicine offered little. Then, through a series of events recovered through alternative medicine and applied neuroscience to becoming an applied neuroscientist, myself."

And ... shortly after that, it was over.

I walked down the three steps from the podium, stood frozen at the end of the stage, and collected a stack of pages with feedback from the judges.

Scarcely believing I presented to this group, I file down the aisle past a sea of kind, encouraging faces and gather a smile from Dr. Julie Silver. I spot my seat and next to it, Kristin, who is beaming. She whispers *I got it! I recorded the whole thing!*

Finally able to breathe again, I nod a polite interest in the next speaker, then dive into the judges' feedback:

"Important book idea."

"Powerful presentation."

"Timely topic."

The ratings were similarly encouraging. I got high marks for organization, relevance of topic, and the presentation itself. Relieved, I put my head down and cried into a tissue.

After the event, I wondered: *Do they tell everyone the same things?* I told Linda I thought maybe the judges were just being nice.

She said: *They ARE nice. But you also did a great job.*

This day was one holy endpoint to a journey, one I want to share with you. I believe my triumph is yours and everyone's who has had a concussion and lingering post-concussion symptoms and felt they couldn't talk about it. It's a triumph for anyone who has felt helpless in the face of being dealt a hand of cards in life that is so not what you wanted. Regardless of what would happen from this point in Boston with my developing book, I had begun to share my story, to say this out loud and to tell medical professionals: there are new and nontraditional tools you may miss that can make a significant difference. Instead of resistance to my message, I felt embraced and supported, like my story mattered. It is a story that, in the end, took me a long time to understand and over two years to write.

Without Permission or Notice

This book describes a journey that took place largely between 2005 and 2010. It is about how an ordinary person, an executive coach and career counselor in private practice, recent author of a first book, on her way home from the gym was waylaid by an accident occurring without permission or notice. In an instant, I suffered one of the 1.5 million concussions that occur in the United States every year.

My car accident that October afternoon was not the worst. Many, many people have suffered so much more. When we hear about concussion and its short and long-term effects, it's most often in the context of catastrophic accidents or professional sports—something remote from what us "regular" people will ever have to confront. Yet head injury and concussion, or traumatic brain injury, is a hidden epidemic with likely greater impact on our lives than you may guess for far less catastrophic injuries.

Most of us have little understanding of concussion and the varied course this injury and its healing may take, let alone the toll it can take on one's interior life and sense of self. Many of us have known someone who's been in an accident and never seemed quite the same: their expectations for life declined, perhaps they pulled back from others, even from themselves. Due to a number of factors, many of them purely luck or coincidence, my path was different.

My Background

Before the 2005 accident, my life was a calendar dotted with client appointments, interviews, presentations, book signings, and looking forward. I am a licensed counselor who has spent more than twenty years studying and coaching others on career and executive development. It's been my joy, my love. My first book called *Back in Control: How to Stay Sane, Productive and Inspired in a Career Transition* (BIC) was the culmination of many secrets about career transition my clients entrusted to me. These insights better prepare people when they have lost a job or find themselves in one that isn't meaningful to them. BIC was a finalist for one of the Nautilus Books Awards—books that help the world become a better place. I am very proud of the wisdom shared by my clients as well as the coaching lessons. Before BIC, my first writing was as a regular contributor on a column in the *Chicago Tribune*'s Sunday newspaper feature called "Insider."

For months after the accident, I wandered through my life, not really being able to see or digest how the accident had affected me. My injury was invisible in that I looked the same, but my life was impacted in rather profound ways I could not see. Traditional medicine provided little structure or resources for my recovery from the lingering symptoms of a moderate concussion. So, through random events, I pursued a path with nontraditional resources and experienced full recovery.

Since story is our best teacher, I will teach you about the amazing tools of my healing and how these have been applied for brain breakthroughs for my clients. These are tools used by professional athletes, executives, and high-performing professionals for peak performance and to deal with everyday issues like anxiety, depression, insomnia, and attention issues.

Giving Words to the Invisible Illness

Writing this book presented many kinds of challenges and rewards. To start, I went through over ten years of journals trying to understand what happened to me, when, and how. My home office looked like a paper storm. I used multiple colors of sticky notes on flip charts posted on my home office walls to sort it out for myself and convey and connect with others around what this time was like. As I put words on paper, I continued to sort out this period of my life to shape this confounding experience into chapters, hoping to adequately describe my journey. Each edit has brought more questions and the necessity to dig deeper to understand, for myself, this confusing period in my life. I was often quizzing my husband and hunting through old calendars, emails, pictures, and whatever I could find to help me understand the impact and sequence. This is brain injury. This is what can happen. If any of this confusion has happened to you, you are not alone. Puzzling my way through this, gaining clarity was hard as well as healing. It showed me what had happened.

Before writing the manuscript, I never wanted to talk much about my injury with people other than my husband. I was never particularly skilled at wrapping words around something I didn't fully or consistently understand. But honestly, I'm also not sure where or how this topic would fit into the conversations I have with most people. When I sprain my ankle and spend a week on crutches, cabs stop for me, people open doors and ask me about it, tell me stories of their sprains and breaks. My moderate concussion left no visible injuries, no radical outward changes in behavior, and few to no words to describe my cognitive deficits and what it's like to lose the anchors in life that helped me be me.

After the accident, my writing life—other than keeping a journal—had essentially stopped. In the occasional writing class or retreat, the unstructured exercises ("write about anything you'd like") almost always landed me in the same place. I would begin to tell the story of my accident and injury, and each time, over and over, it was never to be completed. It was like a boulder in my soul that needed to be released. Now fifteen years later, finally writing my story, pitching it at the Harvard publishing conference, and sharing it with you feels like a way of reclaiming my life. It is a life where I finally understand who I am and how my experiences can bring healing to others.

A Vision for You

In this book, I will tell you my story first as a neighbor or friend and then increasingly as a well-trained professional in the field of applied neuroscience. I will share the random, sometimes humorous, events unfolding the diagnosis and treatment of my brain injury. Humor heals too. I will also share the series of chance events that helped me develop the emotional, physical, social, and spiritual aspects of my life in ways I could have never anticipated. Importantly, I hope to honor my teachers and the relationships that helped shape my life and nurture transformation, giving me a second chance of having a life where I could potentially make a difference. I will share my passion for brain science, which only grew deeper in my recovery and career. Science can change lives, and the cutting edge, brain-based neuroscience tools I describe did just that for me.

I share my story because people need to hear the human stories behind brain trauma and Post-Traumatic Stress Disorder (PTSD), and the tools for healing. It is not only the catastrophic, high-profile stories which can teach us but stories like mine, and clients I have had the privilege of seeing in my role of neuro-therapist, counselor, or executive coach.

This book called *Brain Dance,* embodies the hope and spirit of a whole new era of brain science, which holds promise for mitigating the effects of brain disorders. But also, combined with the ancient wisdom of spiritual practices in the Buddhist tradition, *Brain Dance* fortifies the promise of expanding our human potential through self-regulation of emotions and experiencing joy. This expansion will allow us to act in more skillful, resourceful, and compassionate ways toward our employees, children, partners, and co-workers

True challenges make us stronger and clearer about who we are. I hope my story helps you become more informed, stronger, and clearer in your own life and more courageous about trusting your intuition when events happen that change everything without notice or permission. These events may include a pandemic, the death of loved ones, as well as car accidents. My wish is that you will think about your life differently—especially your brain—and be more mindful of how your brain is working, and what you are doing to take care of it. I trust that the tools and knowledge about physical and psychological transformations will assure you that even when you feel out of control, there are things you can do to change yourself and create better outcomes in life.

My wish is that you will view science as our friend and the brain as this magnificent human organ worthy of our great respect. Many of our social maladies are likely to be improved by optimal brain care for all. And, if you find yourself in a situation in which you can help someone who needs a second chance to learn and grow, that you will do that.

These events are based on my personal recall, which may not be shared by others. Some names and places have been changed; any references to clients and patients are all based on composites, rather than a single case, with any personally identifying details altered to protect their privacy. My goal is to share my emotional truth of a period of time and events that changed my life. And, in so doing, it hopefully help yours or that of someone you love.

So, let's go.

Chapter 1:

In an Instant

Sunday Afternoon

I popped my head through the top of my super-sized sweatshirt, pulled the soft, clean fabric over my sweaty black leotard, and bounced over to get my car from the health club's valet. My favorite attendant flashed me a big smile, grabbed my keys from a glittery wall collection of others, and then came back with my ride. Fall is my favorite season in Chicago, and I've always loved Sundays. It's the day I take care of me. But that day, October 23, 2005, was even more special.

Six weeks after minor surgery and not being able to put full weight on my right foot to do the dance to drive my stick shift car, today was the day. I was finally able to travel to the city alone and work out. I felt strong and independent going solo. My workout was invigorating. I had challenged myself and felt good about my body. A good sweat is the best reward.

When I left my health club, it was misty outside. Despite the rain, the 290 Expressway was clear, so my nine-mile drive from downtown Chicago to my home in Oak Park started smoothly. With my two feet peddling the clutch and accelerator in smooth harmony, I zoomed along on a surface that felt flawless.

I exited the expressway and turned right onto Austin Boulevard, going north and stopped at the first light. Having lived in the Village of Oak Park for over twenty years, I sat there like I had a hundred thousand times before. Listening to the Dixie Chicks in my little gray Saab, I tapped on the steering wheel to the beat and waited for the light to change. I was readying for the tedious path through the one-way, narrow residential streets from the expressway to my home in the center of the Village.

Like tens of thousands of people, I work in the city and live in a nearby suburb. Oak Park is the proud, nearest suburb due west from the city of Chicago. Its claim to fame is being the original home of Frank Lloyd Wright, the father of modern architecture, and the birthplace of Ernest Hemingway. These facts universally emerge in conversations within the first two minutes when proud Oak Parkers talk with visitors. Shaped like a postage stamp of six square miles, Oak Park Village has over 54,000 residents.

As I was singing along in my car, I saw a dark blue sedan on my left coming from Harrison Avenue onto Austin at the light where I was sitting. The car should have been rounding the corner, but it was moving too fast to make this hard-right turn onto the misty street.

Instead, everything seemed to slow down. It was unthinkable, but the sedan seemed to be coming right at me. *What?!*

Car accidents happen millions of times a day, and yet, we never think one will ever actually happen to us. In slow motion, the car drove toward mine. *This is happening. But it can't be happening. It can't. I can manage this. I can manage this,* I thought to myself then tilt, loud sound, *why didn't he stop, cars always stop...* I saw the driver's face as his car slid into my driver's side front bumper. Loud crash. It was not believable. My front fender collapsed, and the hood bowed upon impact. My sweet little car became one of those crushed cars following a wreck. And I was in it.

It happened in an instant, just like a million instants we all have had. And in that instant, without warning or permission, my life changed in small and large ways, some of which I wouldn't realize the enormity of for months, and others in ways that were immediate and could never be fully undone.

After impact, the way the scene unfolded is like a collage in my memory. I remember calling the Chicago police at 9-1-1 and telling them I was in an accident. My voice quivered. It was hard to get the words out on the phone, and then, just like in some wacky commercial, an operator told me I had the wrong number—to hang up and call a different number.

What?... Wait... Are you serious?

I was baffled. Austin Avenue divides Chicago and Oak Park. That fact had never really mattered before in my life. But sitting in the intersection, I learned I had to contact the correct emergency services to get help, and I'm not sure either side of the road wanted to claim me. It was all way too confusing for my brain. People looked at me through the front and side windows, asked me if I was okay, and would I get out of the car. They wanted to move me and get my car out of the intersection. I kept dialing numbers.

I had no cuts or bruises because my head hadn't hit the steering wheel, although it had jolted forward with the impact. Because the other driver had hit my car from the side, the front airbags, the only ones I had, didn't deploy. People asked me how I was, and I said I didn't know. I didn't know how I felt. I remember looking into the mirror to see if I was okay, which didn't help. It was confusing.

In a crisis, many people know we have instinctual response of "fight or flight," but there is also a third mode of response some of us exhibit, and that is "freeze." I felt emotionally frozen, unable to digest things well or make decisions.

Almost without awareness, flashing lights appeared, an ambulance arrived, and I was fielding questions from paramedics. I must have said my head hurt because as a precaution in case I had injured my neck or spine, the ambulance EMT put my head in a square block so I could not move my neck or spine. They strapped me to a narrow board to maneuver me onto a gurney into the ambulance. As they lifted me toward the ambulance, a wave of nausea came over me. In the middle of the intersection, able only to move my eyes, I said weakly, "I feel like I'm going to throw up."

This was clearly not what the burly EMT wanted to hear. In a rather pissed-off tone, he said, "We just got you strapped up here and can't easily stand you up." Translation: "No way, lady, you're wrecking our plan here!"

I swallowed hard and tried to forget how I felt.

The Emergency Room

We got to the ER with my head still strapped into the block. My husband Gary was there by the time the ambulance arrived. He appeared efficient, like he could and wanted to take care of the things that were happening, but with radar available only to a wife of over twenty-five years, his vulnerability leaked out. I knew he was panicking, not knowing how I was or why my head was in the block. When he leaned over me on the crash cart, his eyes were intense, soft, and kind, and he was scared.

"You okay, Hon?" he whispered, holding my hand.

"Yes," I replied, not really knowing if I was but wanting him to be.

It was a busy Sunday afternoon in the West Suburban Hospital Emergency Room. I had to keep the head block on for about ninety minutes. I had waves of panic, feeling trapped since I couldn't move anything but my eyes. I tried not to think about how helpless I felt all strapped down and instead just tried to breathe, lay still, and be lighthearted to reassure my husband. I wondered what would happen to me but tried hard not to think about it.

Gary monitored the situation, peeking out of our curtained-off "room" to see when the medical staff would help me. Finally, a dark-haired, middle-aged doctor swept in with an air of efficiency and did a quick exam. He flashed a tiny light into my eyes and asked me to track it as he moved it up, down, and across. He said there was no concussion, unstrapped me from the block, told me I could go home, and to take it easy and follow up with my doctor the next day. The exam was that quick.

My head and neck felt thick, and a little tingly; I found myself only moving my eyes like I still had that block on my head. I hadn't had a concussion that I remembered, although I was in a significant car accident as a teen. But that was so long ago I remembered little about it. I was hoping to be back to business as usual upon discharge, but it didn't quite feel that way. Not quite. I felt disoriented by the whole situation and was grateful to put my hand in my husband's and leave the busy, crazy hospital.

The Morning After

My husband stayed home from work the next day and drove us to my doctor's office in River Forest, about two miles away. I'll never forget that morning since I went from thinking all was well—that contented feeling you have after deep sleep as you come back to life—to quickly realizing I was unable to tolerate sunlight. The light felt sharp, like something was poking my eyes. I mostly kept them closed during the drive. Sounds were overwhelming—small things like doors closing and street traffic were disturbing to me. Riding in the car, bumps in the road I would have never noticed hurt my body—I kept wishing my husband would roll over them more carefully, but that felt too complicated to put into words. The stopping and going was jarring. I felt like I was made of broken glass.

My doctor was kind, and her staff arranged for me to be examined in a dark room. I laid still and quiet on the table, unlike my generally chatty self. I felt nauseous and overwhelmed by the movement of people around me, the smell of antiseptic—basically everything.

I loved my doctor, Dr. Susan Locke. In grade school, some students get attached to their teachers, hated vacations being away from them, brought them flowers, etc. Other kids didn't care that much at all about their teachers. I cared. Coming from a family in which eight children shared our two parents, it's not surprising my teachers picked up some of the slack. They always made a huge impact on my life—good and bad. I was much happier if they believed in and supported me. Similarly, as an adult, having a kind, smart, and honest doctor made a big difference to me, and Dr. Susan Locke was all that good stuff and more.

After her careful flashlight exam and several questions, she said I had a moderate concussion and told me to take it easy, rest, and take fluids. She also wrote a physical therapy (PT) prescription for whiplash (neck sprain) since my head had been jolted forward and then back. The PT would help the soft tissue injury of my neck and back. I felt she saw and understood me. I got the truth and had a plan. Things would be okay.

While I knew the word concussion, I really didn't know what was in store for me. Even though my symptoms had blossomed since my stint in the emergency room, it seemed the ER doctor had dismissed the possibility of a head injury. Warning us to be on the lookout for delayed symptoms would have been helpful. While our cartoon wisdom of concussion is that when bonked on the head, we see stars and feel dizzy, shake it off, and keep running, in real life, there is growing awareness that perception is incorrect. I was fortunate my husband had taken time off to be available the day after the accident and could drive me.

On Concussion and Being a Baby

In situations we haven't experienced before, like a car accident, head bump, or other trauma, we naturally rely on others, especially professionals. They can help us understand ourselves and how to interpret what's going on and how to proceed. I have met so many people who have been in an auto accident and think there is something wrong with them but don't follow up. Either their doctor didn't suggest that or diagnose a concussion. People who aren't warned could easily try to brush off any delayed symptoms later, believing they don't warrant medical care. They want to ignore their symptoms or, if they do notice them, don't seek help because they don't want to be "a baby." This appears especially true for busy parents; they feel their children should come first, and it would be "selfish" to focus on themselves.

If after an accident or injury involving your head, a doctor says you're okay or that you don't have a concussion, but you don't feel well then or later, don't stop there. Get a second opinion. Doctors are human and can make mistakes, lack knowledge or awareness, or do only the minimum to focus on patients with more life-threatening issues. In many hospital systems, the pressure placed on physicians can be extraordinarily high. But that doesn't mean your symptoms aren't real or don't matter. Understanding concussion and how and when it happens, and its impact is a relatively new area of medicine.

The word concussion comes from the Latin *concutere*, which means "to shake violently." It is a mild traumatic brain injury that can occur after an impact to the head. This could be from a blow to the head, the motion of shaking it (as in "shaken baby syndrome"), or otherwise having the head jolted sharply back and forth.

Anatomy of a Concussion

The brain is made of a gelatinous substance containing trillions of neurons (nerve cells) and is surrounded by fluid—cranial spinal fluid—to cushion it. Upon impact, these neuronal connections get stretched and can be damaged. Impact, either from an outside blow or inside movement, can cause the brain to become bruised and swollen and, therefore, not function well.

While a concussion, or mild traumatic brain injury, is, by definition, not life-threatening, it can result in short- and long-term symptoms that can significantly impact the individual's life.[1] Some would agree the long-term effects of repeated concussions are life-threatening to the injured individual as well as potentially to others around them due to problems with anger, rage, impulse control, and judgment.

Dr. Bennet Omalu Takes on the National Football League

In case you missed the book *Concussion* by Jeanne Marie Laskas or the movie *Concussion* based on it, starring Will Smith, tune in: The

---

1   https://www.emedicinehealth.com/concussion/article_em.htm

concussion conversation became most prominent when, in 2002, Nigerian forensic pathologist Dr. Bennet Omalu was perplexed with why so many professional football players committed suicide or died such early, devastating deaths. As some of the players retired, they showed vexing patterns of cognitive and mood disorders, brain degeneration resulting in dementia, depression, and bouts of anger. By studying the brain tissue donated post-mortem by players, Dr. Omalu found encompassing and shocking changes in the brain structure that he termed Chronic Traumatic Encephalopathy (CTE). These brains were entangled with excess brain protein called Tau, which shut down their ability to function. While living, these players were paid millions for their skills; leaving the field, they often struggled with life and died early. After years of trying to get the NFL to acknowledge and study the impact of repeated concussions, the truth finally was acknowledged, leaving scientists and health professionals to better understand what concussion is and does to the brain.

Even over the last three to five years, we have seen much more research about the impact of blows to the head, and parents much less likely to want their children to be involved in sports that result in such an impact on the brain. Studies show that even high school football players can show early signs of CTE. Soccer players and other athletes also have shown evidence of brain disease resulting from brain and body impact.

Concussion Facts and Myths

A lot has changed during the last fourteen years about our knowledge of concussion and how to treat it, yet some important myths remain. To address these:

- You don't need to be a football player to get a concussion. Low-contact sports, car accidents, and falls or bumps can also cause injury. Players of other sports like soccer, hockey, and polo can also be vulnerable, as well as if you have ever fallen off a swing, bumped your head on a shelf, had someone open a door in your face, had a car accident, or fallen on the ice. Any of those situations and more could result in a concussion.

- ✓ You don't need to hit your head or lose consciousness for you to have a concussion. You can get a concussion without knowing it.
- ✓ Brain injury can happen without a concussion. Repeated blows to the head can cause it or even having your head jolted back and forth without being hit.
- ✓ Even high school football players who have had repeated head hits but never a concussion can show signs of brain injury and early evidence of CTE.
- ✓ Brain injuries can be cumulative, with subsequent ones taking longer to heal.

The signs of a concussion can become apparent immediately or days later. That's likely why it's hard to diagnose. Symptoms can be subtle and resolve in the short-term, or they can be more pronounced and linger for weeks, months, or years depending on several factors.

While some of my symptoms were more obvious over time, others prevented me from truly understanding any of this impact for myself. At the time, this stealthy and under-rated injury tricked me into thinking I was okay when I really wasn't.

In writing this book, I came to appreciate a symptom of brain injury seldom discussed in the literature. That will be pivotal to understanding my story and no doubt that of many other walking wounded with head injuries. I'll tell you more about this as my story unfolds.

Chapter 2:

Wonder Woman... Almost

The Long-Awaited Test

I got past those first few days after the accident with a lot of rest. The following Sunday, I had a Tae Kwon Do (TKD) test for a mid-level belt. I had studied TKD for six years. I knew my forms for this next level and assured my teacher I would feel better by the test date. To be honest, it seemed sort of absurd to go ahead with the test, like someone should have stopped me from thinking it was okay so soon after the accident. But there is also this undefined space around injuries and illness where sometimes doing the normal things, not focusing on pain or symptoms, is absolutely the best thing. My doctor continued to say, "See how you feel." The TKD exams weren't held that often. I had been preparing for months, and I really wanted to get the next level belt. I took things easy that week and planned on going to the test.

My husband drove us in his car, as mine was at the shop where they said it would be for several weeks. The test was held at a gym in Evanston, a suburb north of Chicago. I was excited and wanted to do well. The foot surgery had removed a small but painful cyst on the top of my right foot. It had healed beautifully, and the podiatrist said I earned an "A" for my diligence in keeping up my strength, balance, and overall fitness. Naturally, I was anxious about the test, but what happened is not something that I would have ever predicted.

A belt test involves several hurdles, and many students from different levels were testing that day. To start, we lined up, and the judges shouted commands, putting us through sequences of punches, kicks, and hits while standing together. I successfully executed the first few moves. The next sequence was a step and a punch; I had to step backward and tap my foot behind me. Easy enough: these sequences are the bread and butter of the class warm-up three times a week. The goal was to execute them with perfect form, strength, and precision. Hours and hours of training over a year had prepared me for this moment. Although I looked the part in my crisp white kimono-wrap gee (uniform) tied at the waist by my purple belt, there was one problem: I could not do the move. I could not get my body to take that step backward and punch at the same time.

I stared at this nice judge who seemed to believe in me. The move was certainly something I knew I could do. It was easy. But not now since... I was stuck. I felt perplexed, awkward, and embarrassed like a bumbling little kid unable to manage her body.

That seemed like a fluke, and no one reacted that I could see. I was surprised to be unable to do such a simple maneuver. Though flustered, I went through the rest of the commands in front of the judges. Luckily, there wasn't much left of that part of the test.

Next was two-on-one sparring, with me being the "one" against two senior (black belt) students. My head felt a little fragile as I snapped on my soft helmet and sparring body gear. Even though sparring (fighting) was my favorite activity of all time, the students said they'd go easy on me. That seemed unnecessary because throughout my history in class I was generally fearless and strategic. I wasn't the best in the class by any means, but I was calm and relentless. I had spent hours in class sparring with students of all levels and loved navigating the interdependent dance, looking for the opportunity to score the perfect (air) punch. It was a noncontact activity, although sometimes with unskilled students, in the heat of the moment, a few punches would land. The senior students I was assigned for the test had never sparred with me. They were careful, giving me a wide berth with no close punches or fast moves. They were being nice, which I didn't expect or even want. I was disappointed they seemed to be coddling me a bit. Sparring was my pride. Despite being a little unnerved about the weird step sequence earlier, I felt in control and didn't want to be treated special because I was a "girl." I wasn't thinking about the recent car accident at all. The "careful" sparring wasn't very satisfying since we barely moved around that much, but I made it through without errors or missteps.

Wonder Woman Required

The last hurdle of the belt test was breaking boards with both my elbows and a front leg kick. I was a little nervous at that point because we had never practiced much with real boards in class, and the previous activities hadn't gone quite as I would have planned. Two people held boards on each of my sides at the height of my elbows, and one held a board in front of me.

I walked up to the center of the stage and took my position humbly but as proud as any tall, thin, and delicate-looking woman would be in a situation like that. I was surrounded by senior students, mostly males, in front of a small audience of parents, fellow students, and my husband. I folded my hands together in a wide prayer position, just above my heart.

The next thing I heard was myself yelling, "HEY!" at the top of my lungs, shattering the silence in the gym. The Key-Up (yell) is part of the move—the louder, the better. My elbows flew up and then out. I swiftly elbowed the boards to each side, cracking them one by one. All you could hear in the gym was the cracking of the boards, the huge gasp of a woman in the audience, and then loud applause. It was a superwoman moment, quickly followed by a front kick that did not break the board. I was disappointed about the last part, but the woman's gasp, audience applause, and my feeling of momentary strength was epic. I will never, ever, forget that scene and the emotional snapshot of centered strength, power, and humility. I had hoped I would have felt that way for the whole exam, which was all well within my capabilities. At least, I had thought it was.

When the scores were tallied, I had passed conditionally, but I didn't feel as if I had done my best. At some point soon, I needed to re-demonstrate some of the forms I was unable to perform—those easy ones. Doing poorly had seemed inconceivable to me because I had worked so hard to prepare. Students train for months before the teacher will even let them test. I'm not sure why or how I passed. The judges reassured me that my legs getting stuck in the first sequence was simply because I was nervous. But to me, that was like saying someone who forgot how to walk was probably nervous.

The Roots of My Passion

It's important to tell you what doing all this meant to me. I love TKD. It's a spiritual practice for me. I would find myself and even a connection to my ancestors in practicing the repetitive, powerful movements. It's like poetry for my body, fostering a strength and confidence I never had before. I grew up in a household with an often frustrated and overwhelmed mother with eight children who ruled with a paddle and an iron fist. A complex woman of many strengths, she treated us the way she had been treated, no doubt. I loved my mom, and she did many kind things. But I often felt helpless and scared for myself and my siblings on her bad days.

With the level of skill I had mastered in TKD, I exceeded my dream of being capable of protecting myself. It satisfied my "inner child." I also felt as if I could protect other people if I ever had to, like my husband on the CTA (Chicago Transit Authority) Green Line traveling to and from Chicago's Loop to our home in the suburbs. Like in most big cities, thousands of us take public transportation routinely, but it's not always safe. If anything ever threatened my safety, I had a weapon I could use. Myself.

My injury challenge was unfolding around the same time as Hurricane Katrina hit, displacing thousands of people, many of whom were evacuated to unsafe places where they were assaulted and victimized. I would imagine myself being a warrior for them, going down to New Orleans to help protect the hurricane refugees and teach them how to protect themselves. I imagined putting the kids staying in the football stadium in a big circle and teaching them moves and how to be strong in the face of challenge.

Similarly, to motivate myself, I would replay in my head the airplane cabin scenes of the 9/11 hijackings and murder of the United and American Airlines flight attendants and passengers. For many years, my husband worked for a major airline, and we had the privilege of traveling often to visit my husband's extended family on the West Coast. Airplane cabins felt like sanctuaries for peaceful moments, and they were a constant fixture in my life. The attacks were an assault on that personal sense of peace and safety.

Perhaps like many martial artists, I suppose, I replayed these hijacking scenes over and over in my head. I imagined how I might have helped disarm the hijackers and save lives.

My doctor knew I loved Tae Kwon Do and believed the movement would also help me heal and regain a sense of competence and balance. After the belt test, she suggested taking a couple of weeks off from class and then seeing how I felt going back.

Sounded good, right?

Chapter 3:

That Undefined Space

"You Already Told Me..."

Sidelined for a couple of weeks, I was decked out in my crisp white Tae Kwon Do uniform, sitting on the hardwood floor at the side of the large room watching the class. This is the custom if you can't participate because of an injury or you've entered the room after class has started. It's like sitting in the dugout in baseball or on the bench in basketball.

I leaned over to whisper to a senior student next to me who was recovering from ankle surgery. "I can't participate for a couple of weeks because I was in an accident and have a head and neck injury," I said.

He lifted his chin and looked me in the eyes. "You already told me that same thing just a second ago. You told me that EXACT same thing!"

He moved back and stared straight ahead for the rest of class. That smarted since I thought he was a cool guy, and I never had much of an opportunity to talk with him in class. The club was full of cool guys – local and some national celebrities. However, most people were super nice, even if this guy wasn't.

Part of me knew I had repeated myself. But another part of me didn't know and trusted that I wouldn't have done something weird like that. So, I tried not to give it much more thought. The part of me that knew I had repeated myself felt unsettled, but I assured myself the moment would pass.

At the same time, I felt like I shouldn't be there and instead should be at home. I didn't know how to act. My head felt fragile. It was like I had to hold my head just right, or it would fall off. I couldn't turn it completely, and my neck was sore. Things felt slightly off-kilter, and like everything was moving fast around me. I thought I would feel better soon. It was as if someone should have told me I shouldn't be there, like if you go to work when you're sick and your boss just sends you home. But no one knew how I felt, so how could they? I was just working my way through something that was undefined, my head and neck injury, thinking that trying to keep to my schedule was the best thing.

Your Brain Holds Back

Over the next weeks, I wanted to rally, and above all, just be okay and go on with my life. But it didn't work out that way. Life became strange, although I didn't put the pieces together at the time.

The brain is our driver. It's hard when it's not a reliable navigator. And the trickiest thing is that your brain, even when it's not okay, may still try to convince you that it is.

It's a trouper and does its best. It's like a car GPS that resets when you don't follow its instructions. It doesn't have a tantrum and say:

"Now that you have messed this drive up and made the wrong turn, go back and do it over!" Instead, it lets you make a wrong turn and then calmly says, "Resetting, drive straight ahead and turn left at the next street."

With a calm, redirecting GPS voice, you can't tell you've even screwed up. Even though you might have made the biggest driving route mistake you could possibly imagine, taking you way out of your way and incurring many more miles, the GPS simply says what to do next.

The brain navigator does the same thing. It doesn't let on that you are screwed, that your balance, body coordination, and short-term memory now suck, that you have the concentration of a fruit fly. It just keeps calmly redirecting you, trying its best with whatever resiliency, however damaged, it has. At least, this is what mine did. My brain's navigation of what was happening and what I needed to do for myself wasn't the best, but I couldn't see that. Hence, for example, I was there in TKD class, telling the senior student next to me over and over about my accident.

I wanted to be the same old me and stay with my routine, but as time passed, the changes in my brain were making my life more and more difficult—something even I could see.

But I persisted. I just wanted to be okay. Like I was before.

Unreliable Navigation and Confusing Times

In mid-November, three weeks after my car accident, I decided to take six weeks off from class and from my executive coaching and career counseling private practice. It wasn't that I had any clear perspective on what was happening to me or how I was functioning or that anyone suggested it. But I felt like nothing I tried to do turned out well, and I needed a break. I had never taken a six-week break from work in my whole life. My doctor approved. I always felt reassured when I saw her but didn't have the impression there was more to do to promote healing or more tests I should be taking. I believed she was concerned about me. I trusted her and still do. Her approach seemed to be that we'd "wait and see" and that I'd be okay at some point soon.

Looking back, I can see how my emotions were all over the place. I often fought with my therapist (all coaches have their own coach or therapist) about silly things around appointment reschedules or who said what in conversations. Things on my "to-do" list never got done, day after day. I often lost my keys, jackets, and other things. I had attention deficit disorder (ADD) before the accident. After it, all my usual struggles were amped up. I went out to meet a friend and discovered my top was inside out or I had the wrong day—those kinds of things. Self-employed, I felt too overwhelmed to do much more than to keep my small coaching practice going. It was important for me to do a good job with the work I took on. I certainly didn't feel strong enough to market my business or pursue public speaking engagements like I had done to promote my book. Instead, I spent a lot of time on the Internet—my brain loved to focus on small details, and I would get lost in online rabbit holes for hours.

In daily life, my focus and self-awareness seemed banished, replaced by faint shadows and increasingly unreliable navigation. Only I didn't know it. One example: Starting the summer before the accident, a graduate student who had read my book on career development contacted me. She said she loved the book and wanted me to supervise her for an internship that would start in January. Over the next months, we went back and forth, pinning down the school requirements and paperwork before meeting in person in early December. When she was arranging this meeting, I told her about the accident but assured her I would be feeling better soon. We met, and everything seemed fine: She had such energy, enthusiasm, and great ideas for working together. Overall, she seemed like a fabulous person. But after our meeting, I never saw or heard from her again. In the dense sea of my thinking, I could never figure that out. Months passed, and somehow, I kept expecting to hear from her. Well, when I thought about it.

With little else on my plate, I wanted to find a way of moving forward, to see some positive movement in some part of my life. The co-author of a writing project we had started months earlier suddenly dropped off the face of the earth and never returned a phone call. I knew she had taken a new job and was busy but to n-e-v-e-r call me back? Ever? I can just remember how vulnerable I felt calling her the very last time, after several attempts, and leaving a voicemail trying to sound upbeat and not upset, asking her to please call me. My husband was in the car, driving me to the office. It was somehow this grasp at feeling I had something positive going on in my life. But she never called back. For years I dropped out of the professional groups we had both belonged to, so it was over ten years before our paths crossed again. Talk about awkward.

It was a confusing time. I didn't understand it. I didn't have the vocabulary to identify—let alone explain—what was happening to me. Overall, my gut feeling was that I needed to stop—to stop what I was doing overall. Not that I understood that I was injured or how it was affecting me and how I presented myself or worked; I just felt like nothing worked.

Hopefully, people will learn from my story and recognize some of the markers of this kind of injury, and help others make decisions like taking a break much earlier and longer, if needed. If you are injured, you will be more likely to recognize the confusion, forgetfulness, increased emotional vulnerability and reactivity, disorganization, and short-term memory issues in yourself. And, you will also tell your doctor or health care team so you can get help.

Everyone reacts to concussion differently, but the more you know about these more subtle yet life-changing symptoms, the better.

Physical Therapy Fortune and Failure

My doctor had prescribed physical therapy (PT) for my head and neck injuries. I believe that PT should be available to everyone because building strength and mobility is a great way to get past bodily pain. People who pass on this option if it is available to them do themselves a serious injustice.

I was lucky because the PT facility we found was one of the best in the city. Its therapists treated the dancers in Chicago's high-profile companies, political figures, and professional athletes. One afternoon, as I looked around at all the patients in the gym treatment room, I realized I was the only one there without an entourage or a handler nearby. Funny how I just got used to seeing these people day in and day out in their sloppy workout clothes, like me. We struggled earnestly and, at points, shared the humor in the rehab journey with its highs and lows, and the weird and difficult exercises our PTs had us doing in the gym. They were the closest thing I had to new friends—the other patients I saw. Pain and vulnerability create unspoken bonds.

I came in with neck pain, occasional dizziness, balance issues, and an inability to turn my head to one side completely. That kept me from driving, as did the lack of a car. Mine would be in repair for at least six weeks, which was okay with me since I could take the train downtown or ride other places with my husband. Besides, I felt uneasy behind the wheel of a car or even riding in one for that matter.

After the injury, when I did my usual workout on the cross-trainer at the gym, standing pumping my arms back and forth while peddling my feet, I could feel my brain bouncing up and down in my skull. The sensation was weird, uncomfortable, and one I had never felt before, so I stopped doing the cross-trainer. I doubt I mentioned it to my doctor or thought that much about it since I knew I was injured. I just stopped doing that exercise.

Going to PT downtown two to three times a week created a structure and support for staying active when I didn't feel like doing much. It enabled a better shift of my patterns on how to best exercise, like indoor cycling and no cross-trainer. I attended diligently and did my "at home" program the same way. My physical therapist told me I was an "A" student. I can't say enough about the good people who helped me. However, no one could identify or help me understand what had happened to my brain. Not that I noticed at the time. I probably didn't tell the therapists enough about how I felt other than my pain and strength levels.

Those Tiny Needles

Another mainstay of my life during this phase was acupuncture. Those single strands of hair-thin needles placed into my back, head, and neck helped the healing. For me, these treatments began a long time before the accident, and I got regular treatments to keep me healthy. After the accident, I changed my schedule from once per month to twice weekly for a while. The Chinese doctor I see is Dr. Lo, who has rare credentials. He was trained at Northwestern University Medical School in Internal Medicine as well as in China for traditional Chinese medicine. Both of his parents had similar credentials. He's a very careful observer and doesn't talk very much. He analyzed my energy and looked for blocks by having me stick out my tongue, studying its color and coating. He also felt the pulse at my wrist to see if it was "thready," quick, or had other characteristics commonly identified in traditional Eastern medicine. He placed needles along the meridians of the body to unblock the different types of energy that nourish life and let the body heal itself. They have names like gall bladder, heart, and liver meridians. I've always slept better and had less tension and pain after acupuncture. I feel better after acupuncture in some fundamental ways that have no correlations in the language of Western medicine. Chinese medicine can be powerful and highly recommended when done by well-trained providers.

I think my young, athletic PT initially had doubts about whether or not acupuncture really helped, but in working on my body, she could always tell if I had had acupuncture the day before or that week since the muscles in my neck and back would have fewer spasms and be more mobile and relaxed.

Me and the Green Shirts

During my six-week leave in late 2005, volunteer work seemed like a great idea. I signed up for a day at the Greater Chicago Food Depository a few days before Christmas. Several acquaintances from a professional organization had organized the outing, and while I didn't know these people well, I was eager to engage with the outside world again for a worthwhile cause. My husband dropped me off, and I found my group. I remember looking at these people, thinking they looked like the people I knew, only they were dustier somehow, and slightly older versions of themselves. They were all smiling, retired, and happy to be out helping, but I felt too young to be doing volunteer work during a workday. They were terribly kind but said things like: "What are you doing here? How's your book going?"

I also found myself surprisingly self-conscious about my weight for the first time in many years. I grew up in a thin family where I was the only one of three girls who struggled with weight as a young adult. It wasn't easy.

My recent weight gain wasn't something I'd realized until that day. Despite PT, my level of exercise was nowhere near what it had been. Since the accident, I had put on weight and suddenly felt like a chubby and denser version of myself. It undermined any confidence I had in a rather fundamental way, leaving me feeling like the "fat sister." It reminded me of when I first started struggling with my weight. I had gone away to college and gained twenty pounds. It was brutal to look so different from my former self and my sisters. When my younger sister first saw me, she laughed so hard she fell down backward on the bed. It wasn't funny to me. Pretty painful. My eating challenges had been addressed in the years that followed. I felt like I was a normal size for myself with normal eating habits. However, after the accident, that had somehow disappeared.

One section of the Depository warehouse was sectioned off to create a room for sorting small cereal boxes from a bin. We wore masks. A large plastic strip door curtain enclosed the area where we worked. Within five minutes, my face and throat started swelling, and I struggled to take full breaths. Apparently, little particles of cereal escaped into the air of this confined area. I tried to stay, but as hard as it was to believe, I could hardly breathe.

Looking back, I realize how this happened. When the brain and nervous system encounter trauma, sensitivities to different foods or airborne environmental elements can occur. Resilience is lower. Things previously neutral can become toxic to the body. If you have a head injury, it's important to clean up your diet and stick to whole foods (vegetables, good fats, and proteins) since your brain needs energy to repair itself. Sometimes sensitivity to foods or your environment may change at least temporarily. I'll talk more about this later.

My reaction surprised me and added to my developing sense of strangeness about the day. I pulled back from the huddle of my colleagues and slipped out between the heavy plastic strips.

The Food Depository floor manager said I could join another group that had a project in the open area of the floor. The job entailed selecting materials from a conveyor belt to fill boxes with the right combination of goods. The new workgroup came from a local bank. They all had on matching green shirts imprinted with their bank logo.

I loved this manual work. It felt so good to move and do something easy. Growing up, I was always a busy kid working on something like helping my mom pick and can vegetables in the summer with my brothers and sisters, twirling my baton outside for hours, and just "doing things." Filling the boxes demanded a certain group coordination to ensure all the correct parts were put together, that each person had enough stock to do his or her part. I took over leading the effort and enjoyed helping the team get in sync. I felt decisive and direct with my body language. I loved that the team came to rely on me for direction. After having been sidelined from my normal life and not feeling all that skillful, I was ready to go to work and do something real. Being with people, especially in new relationships, felt great. I was happy in my new group.

At the end of the day, a department head from the green shirt company gave a little speech about the food bank. The group started to leave when someone said they were going to do a group photo. I was excited to be in the picture. I followed the people I had been working closest with to where they were organizing the photo.

"Only people in the green shirts in the picture," a man said as he looked to the department head.

Somehow this comment and the speaker's frustrated tone logged in my memory though I didn't understand what was happening at the time. I felt a little left out, but nothing major. After the photo, the rest of the group was still friendly, and it had been fun working together. It was still a great experience because I hadn't been out that much, and I finally felt like I could do something valuable. I was joyous.

As I was walking out, I started talking with the lead manager, mentioned my background in organizational development, and said, "This would be a great exercise for team-building!"

I was oblivious to the fact that the team manager had been trying to do exactly this—build his team. I had missed the cues and somehow taken over the role of team leader instead of someone from their actual team. I was entirely oblivious. To this day, I feel embarrassed to even think about it. Oy. I hope this memory will be funnier someday soon.

Concussion = The Expensive Smaller Plate

If you had asked me how I felt during this time, I would have said, "Fine!" I had headaches sometimes, and certain head movements made me feel nauseous, but these symptoms seemed transient. In TKD and exercise classes, I couldn't do fast turns or spin without struggling with balance and feeling dizzy. So, I avoided any moves involving spinning and turning.

Overall, it was like having a much smaller plate in life. Before, I had a decent-sized plate with friends, activities, commitments, and events to look forward to. But after the accident, my capacity shrunk. Things fell off that I would have never dreamed would. There were appointments or tasks I had to follow up on. I would be late and sometimes left tasks unfinished. This was totally unlike me, especially with important things.

I had an awareness of this "small-plate" experience at the time but a rather dulled reaction to it. That's just the way my life was then. I could see that much. But it was also sort of inconceivable and like watching a train wreck in very slow motion without sound. I didn't recognize any connection between all this and my head injury.

For example, a company was interested in developing a corporate training program based on the principles in the book I had just written. What an amazing and potentially lucrative situation—every author's dream. After taking many small steps to get to that point, I had to meet and collaborate in person with company executives about the details. I was no more prepared for this than for a ride to the moon. Cognitively, it was far beyond anything I could think through. This opportunity fell off my shrinking plate.

How could I possibly let such an important and expanded recognition of my work slip away? When I think back on what the executives were asking for, their requests weren't unusual. To a clear, capable mind, their requests were reasonable.

I remember talking with my therapist about how I just couldn't send them one more email to pin down this opportunity and move forward. They were eager and excited but seemed to need so much information and follow-up. I just couldn't do it. He looked at me, stroked his speckled beard, and said, "How do you feel about that?" It was the predictable "therapist as impartial observer" response.

Given that he is a medical doctor, and I had recently had a moderate concussion, I would have hoped for a much different and better response. Now, there are more resources for people with concussions so that they don't make major decisions while injured even if they can't see or aren't aware of their current limitations. My primary care doctor was my rock during this journey when I saw her and could articulate what was going on. I felt like she cared, and that made all the difference in my world. Yet, there was and still is a dearth of understanding and resources for the everyday person who has a concussion.

It's possible these professionals were more proactive than I am describing. They may have structured my concussion recovery and suggested limiting screen time and balancing rest and activity and diet. Perhaps I didn't remember receiving this advice. However, I don't think so, and my husband, who has been the greatest reality-tester for me in writing this book, doesn't remember it that way either. Concussions weren't a focus ten-plus years ago. Many health care providers are more knowledgeable and proactive now, but there is still room for awareness and studies on best protocols for concussion and post-concussion treatment.

The biggest challenge with my brain injury was not understanding how my functioning was impaired. I knew some things were sliding.

The biggest example: We had invested a lot in the birth of my book. It had been my calling, my baby, and I felt it would help many people. My husband had even taken an early retirement to find a publisher for it. There was no part of me, though, that could even grasp—let alone reverse—the dismantling of the life my husband and I had worked so hard to create.

A Stroke of Insight?

In 2008, three years after my accident, the book, *My Stroke of Insight, A Brain Scientist's Personal Journey,* came out. This book documents a neuroscientist's observations about the devastation of her own stroke. People who knew about my injury said, "Diane, this must be how you felt." I'm grateful for the book and the brave Dr. Jill Bolte Taylor for sharing her experience. It helped people find a way to begin to address this type of injury.

However, all brain injuries are not alike. Dr. Bolte Taylor had a stroke on one side of her brain while the other side was intact. Concussions, however, are from diffuse axonal injury (DAI) from the brain's movement in the skull, like shaken baby syndrome. The whole brain can be affected. The changes are more subtle and global, often with a lack of awareness that they're happening. It wasn't until I was well into my recovery that I could recognize the world I'd created to manage and compensate for my deficits.

My friends later described my affect as overall, I wasn't present. The Diane they knew wasn't quite there. I talked slowly. My world became very small, and after just having written and launched my first book, the contrast was big.

During the book launch, my well-connected publicist arranged many TV and radio interviews for me, including ABC, NBC, and public radio. I would often delight my friends by sharing the where and when details of these interviews. My friends lovingly shared in my excitement around all things book related. After the accident, I rarely spoke about my book. I couldn't see these changes myself. My self-awareness was limited. It's been hard to summarize the subtle and not-so-subtle effects of having a brain injury until you're past it.

It's Spouses Who Suffer

The people closest to us can have the hardest road in many ways. One day shortly after the accident, I recall my husband saying goodbye and leaving the house to do errands. When he kissed my cheek, I was sitting in a straight-backed chair in the living room in front of the long French windows but facing away from them. When he came back three hours later, I was in the same position, staring straight ahead. I hadn't moved. I hadn't even tried to move. I really couldn't do more than sit, content to stare. I was okay if I didn't move. I was better. It was what I needed to do. It's hard even to write this because I can only guess how terrified my poor husband felt. The smart, capable woman he married now just stared. He told me later he was afraid for me for many months. Spouses and all significant others deserve support to manage the stress of an uncertain future, feeling powerless to make a difference, and their own losses resulting from having an impaired partner. While my husband is a hardy, resourceful guy, I wished he had more outside support in dealing with my long, confusing journey in healing my brain.

Inside Mental Deficiency

As a young child, a mental game, almost an obsession, was to look at people and try to understand how it felt inside to be them. Maybe this came from living with a sometimes unpredictable mother whose moods shifted and whose actions had consequences for me. But it's a skill that has served me well as a coach and therapist. At one dim moment shortly after my concussion, I remember thinking I now knew what it felt like to be Doogie, our neighbor from when I was about six or seven years old.

Doogie—short for Douglas—was developmentally delayed and a puzzle to my young mind. He didn't understand things we all could understand. He was slow and spoke loudly with a different rhythm than everyone else. He sometimes had intense emotions over small things. I never understood his experience being trapped in the body he had. I could never make a connection with him. I tried. He was stuck in a language and processing speed all his own. It was a ping of insight, after all these years when Doogie came to mind. I checked this off as solving one of my childhood mysteries. This was the mental state I had been so curious to understand as a child.

I now was slow, unable to keep things in my mind and not lose track of them. But at the same time, I was aware of it being a peaceful state. Being slow wasn't being miserable, just slow. That's surprising, isn't it? Having been on the lower-functioning side, I will never take my mental and physical capacities for granted again or try never to make assumptions about how others feel.

Chapter 4:

But I Love Your Shoes!

Lured by the Shiny M

Around mid-February of 2006, about five months after the accident, I wanted to drive my car again. I could turn my head okay, and I felt ready to get behind the wheel again. That was temporary. It happened one afternoon coming home from PT. I was sitting at a stoplight, relaxed and calm, listening to music when something caught my attention. I found myself staring at this large shiny letter. It was an M, and I was mesmerized, trying to figure out if it looked like a shiny, candy M&M. A honking horn snapped me to attention. I discovered I had drifted into the middle of an intersection without realizing it. I was staring at the shiny front grill of a huge Mack truck across the intersection from me. A big shiny M.

I scared myself—no more driving for a while.

Riding in the car as a passenger wasn't always that fun either. For example, one evening, my husband and I were driving home from Costco on a two-lane road having a perfectly normal conversation, when out of the blue I yelled: "STOPPPPP!" and threw my hands up in front of my face.

"WHAT? WHAT?" Gary said in a panic, looking madly back and forth.

Me: "DIDN'T YOU SEE THAT CAR? HE WAS GOING TO HIT US!"

"NO, HE WASN'T," Gary said. "He was just turning on a green turn light." He exhaled loudly and gripped the steering wheel at ten and two o'clock. "Don't yell at me like that! You scared me. I'm driving."

I wrapped my arms around myself. "Do you think I'm doing this for the fun of it? I can't stop myself. If we're about to be hit, I'm going to tell you."

These heated interactions in the car happened more than once. I honestly didn't realize how this was part of the fabric of our travel lives until my sweet teenaged nephew visited and was sitting in the back seat. I could somehow see our dynamic through his eyes: We are normal people: his Aunt Diane and Uncle Gary, who live in Chicago. Nice people. We are fine and friendly, and I yell now and then whenever I believe someone will be hitting us in our car. So, I'm quirky. Let's not talk about it. I get scared. Enough said.

I had gone back to work in January 2006, only seeing a few clients. My days were filled with going to physical therapy, acupuncture, and some work. I wasn't sure that my physical therapist even thought I had a job. As a coach and psychotherapist, I didn't talk much about my work, certainly not personal details. My life wasn't stressful, and I was starting to enjoy day trading. Yes, I said day trading. It was one of the rabbit holes I'd fallen into on my Internet tours. It made me feel interesting, like I did something... daring. When I talked with my PT about day trading, she didn't say much. There was little conversation. My attempt at having an interesting life didn't seem to work. Reflecting, I'm sure she thought I was crazy. More on that later.

What coaches or psychotherapists trade commodities? It is such a weird hobby, but in 2006's positive financial climate, it was exciting and rewarding. Every trade was a frightening, thrilling decision. I'd put a thousand dollars on a stock to see if it would go up, and I could sell it for more. With every trade, my heart pounded in my ears, and I felt incredibly powerful and helpless at the same time. Powerful in taking on a dare, a real risk. Helpless in that the market is way bigger and more powerful than I am, and money can be gone in an instant. Money gone is money gone. I danced carefully among market ups and downs, staying with my Motley Fool researched picks. This felt like the one area in my life where I was competent. I skimmed websites and read up on what others were saying about the market and specific stocks.

I didn't feel grossly incompetent overall, but instead, I felt like I was waiting for an intangible something, not sure what, before I could think about making goals and moving ahead again with my life. I was still in this undefined space in life, taking care of the moment the best that I could. My identity as a writer-author had collapsed. The book I wrote had fallen off my plate of awareness. I never thought about it for at least a year. It wasn't part of the world I lived in day to day. I kept my life as peaceful as I could. I am grateful for the office arrangement I had during this time that allowed me to use the space as much or as little as I needed. Even if I wasn't seeing clients all the time, having a job helped hold my life together as well. I've always loved my work.

During this time, I kept a personal journal as I had since I was sixteen years old, as well as a gratitude journal. Each day I wrote three things I was grateful for. I watched *The Oprah Winfrey Show* daily. Mental attitude is so important in life, and I was always working on mine. Sure, my life was smaller. I didn't feel like going to professional meetings; I didn't feel strong enough even to consider giving presentations or looking for opportunities to expand my coaching and therapy practice. I was... waiting.

Trading Stocks with Our Retirement Funds

Frightening but true.

As I mentioned, one of the things my injured brain loved to do was study details. Well, obsess and dig deep into things. While my mind seemed incapable of following through on even some basic professional and personal routines of my pre-injury life, I could perversely keep a laser-like focus on the details of endless Internet searches regarding stocks. My mind didn't have much focus for anything else. I loved to get lost in researching companies, analysts' opinions about those companies, profit-earnings ratios, and other financial indices.

When my husband took early retirement to sell my book to a publisher, he rolled over his retirement funds to a large investment and brokerage firm. In my free time—and I had lots—I started to study these accounts. It seemed easy to improve upon the investing my husband's company had done with our 401(k)s. I learned about the Morningstar rating system for funds, with five stars being the best and one the worst, relating to investment returns. I discovered that Gary's money was invested in funds that were all rated one star. I figured it was a real "no brainer" that a fund rated with five stars was much better. So, I did lots of sampling of analyst opinions to find "better" mutual funds and then moved the money into them.

At night, I would research ideas and then prepare orders to execute in his accounts in the morning when the market opened. Then I'd wake up the next morning before the market opened and wonder if I had made the best decisions. I could cancel the orders and change things back in the morning before the orders went to market. It was like practicing buying and selling funds since I had never done it. After a while, I started tracking what would have happened had I left the orders in place and made my purchases. My success rate was impressive. If my orders had executed, our funds would have earned well. In this made-up world of me being an investment fund manager, I was making profitable decisions, even though I wasn't putting the orders through. You see, my husband didn't know I was pretending and planning to move money around in his accounts. Well, to be honest, I did execute some of those orders.

When the company where he worked for many years filed for bankruptcy in 2002, my husband had a catastrophic feeling about our finances. Like thousands of people, the bankruptcy entailed huge financial and emotional losses for us. We struggled to believe we could count on anything, including things he had worked for his whole life. Both his pension and a fund based on an employee ownership plan collapsed. Our future financial stability was a very vulnerable topic. Gary prided himself on taking good care of us financially, and he got the short end of the company's bankruptcy filing.

One evening over dinner, I just couldn't keep the secret a second longer and confessed to my husband about what I had been doing with his retirement accounts—mine were small at that point. After his panic passed, he agreed I could make small, carefully thought out changes in the accounts as long as I told him ahead of time. This was a big step for both of us. Gary didn't know much about investing, so I took this on as my job. Over the years, he's come to call me the "family fund manager." I read a lot and talk to financial representatives whenever I can.

I also day-traded stocks. Day trading means you buy and sell something within the same day. I mainly focused on one stock in the beverage arena. It was the Monster energy drink, then from the Hansen Corporation. I kept to the goal of buying low and selling high and clearing all sales the same day, if possible. The stock was volatile, going up and down dramatically as people discovered, hated, and then loved energy drinks. It was thrilling for me to buy a hundred shares at $75 each and then sell the same hundred-share lot for $82 each. That's a profit of $700. Even though these might seem like small numbers for a real trader, for me, who didn't expect to be making any money trading stocks, it was simply unbelievable. I wasn't very goal-focused in my life, at all. That part of my brain, the frontal lobe with its executive functions, wasn't that engaged. I was obsessed with learning about this.

I also made small trades in my own meager retirement account, and it grew substantially. I now thank the heavens for the Motley Fool newsletter, Jim Cramer, Morningstar ratings, and my hours of obsessive research.

It wasn't as big of a stretch as it may sound. As a career coach, I had worked with several traders from the Chicago Mercantile Exchange. Some of them knew a lot about finance and the market. Others didn't have technical knowledge, but they had their own systems, like astrology, to figure out how and when to bet. All that insight certainly gave me a lot of moxie to venture into trading with only my degrees in psychology. If they could invest their own funds and do well, I certainly could try.

I traded in our accounts in 2006-2007 and made enough money to equal the pay of a part-time job. One of my friends pointed this out to me when I was complaining of feeling like a failure. It was a strange phase of my life because I felt disconnected from the things I loved most and unable to execute anything with a high level of competence, except trading our investments. This aspect of my life went pretty well, objectively. Obsession, which was amplified by the injury, was put to good use. Also, many people who have frontal lobe injuries have subtle (or dramatic) changes in personality. From the car accident impact, my head jolted forward then back, and the brain does too, even though it balances in a pool of gel to cushion that. The front and back of the brain typically suffer impact in these situations, as well as the temporal lobes of the brain, which can scrape within the skull structure. This new hobby was a change from things I knew and required an element of thrill-seeking from risk-taking that didn't fit my previous temperament, although I did love sparring in TKD.

My advice on this is: Please learn a lot before you try day trading at home.

Real Rocks in My Head?!

On the physical side, I was working on neck and back pain and neck mobility. Besides my lack of overall focus and general fogginess (unless I was hyper-focused on something like day trading), I had a persistent problem with dizziness and sometimes headaches. Often in physical therapy, when lying down, the PT would cup my head in her hand, rub the tension out of my neck, and then gently turn my head to increase the range of motion. Each time, I usually felt dizzy and nauseous. Similarly, I felt dizzy when I stood up after lying down, if I bent over and hung my head, or spun around quickly in TKD or elsewhere.

My PT thought talking with a neurologist might be a good idea. My doctor agreed. It was hard to make an appointment, but my doctor's referral got me onto a neurologist's calendar for an appointment two months away. It seemed a long time to wait, but I planned to cancel if the issue resolved before then or if I got another resource. One month later, the neurologist's office called to ask (again) why I was coming in. I explained my symptoms a second time. She canceled my appointment, saying they had more serious cases to treat, the doctor's schedule was full, and they couldn't help me. I was stunned. How could they do that? I eventually adopted everyone else's attitude, including my doctor's: Don't worry, simply work away at getting healthier.

After trying several approaches to help the vertigo, my capable PT came across a technique that involved repositioning the crystals in my ears. It was a technique she had just learned at an out-of-town conference.

Our balance is preserved by crystalline rocks of calcium carbonate in the inner ear, the vestibular system. They are sensitive to gravity and kept in place by a jelly-like membrane. When these rocks or weights are displaced from a blow to the head or jarring shake, they can end up in different locations than they should be. The weights become unbalanced and can cause dizziness.

I was the star of the clinic the day she led me through special exercises as other therapists observed. My PT proudly demonstrated a series of bold maneuvers, like hanging my head off the end of a treatment table while I was lying on my back, turning me upside down, sideways, and every other way you can think of as she situated and resituated my head to move these little rocks. It was awful, but I tried to be brave since people were watching. I ended up feeling dizzy and nauseous, which wasn't supposed to happen, but the protocol was worth trying and certainly gave new meaning to the expression "they have rocks in their head." The dizziness improved only slightly after the treatment and didn't go away completely for months. My PT said it didn't make sense. We proceeded with what we had been doing before her conference.

This Is Me?!

By late March 2006, five months after the accident, I started to put some words and understanding around what was happening to my life. I could see my path was one of going to PT, doing part-time work, TKD, and exercising. I started to understand myself as someone who had been through something, even though it was hard for me to define or talk about it with other people. I never wanted to be anything but okay.

My world had become fairly small. I didn't talk to many people. I just felt absorbed with my own life, my husband, and a few close friends. But very slowly, I began to find the pieces that made sense out of my things and cast it into a story of what had happened to me.

Love Your Shoes!

First, a little background: When we launched *Back in Control* in June of 2004, I had the great honor of having my first signing at the largest independent bookstore in Chicago. It was a wonderful place that hosted many great book events—workshops and signings. I loved the setting, and the people who worked there were great. My publicist, Lissy Peace, arranged it, and we were all so excited.

That evening, an intense storm rolled in. The rain beat down horizontally. We could hardly walk from the car to the store. Umbrellas collapsed and blew away, hair and bags dripped with water. Still, inside the bookstore, the ambiance was incredibly warm. We entered a spacious room with a presenter's area along the right wall, and the rest filled with rows and rows of books, small hanging chimes, and greeting cards. The gentle scent of cinnamon and cloves hung in the air. Small votive candles dotted the shelves near a collection of mystical statues. Norah Jones' "Come Away with Me" played softly. No wonder this was a coveted place to launch a book.

The presentation area in the store's center was filled with people who were warm and interested. Many of my friends came. The evening was all any author could ever possibly dream of—to be surrounded by wisdom and love while sharing my work with the uncompromising goal of helping people. It was fantastic. We also sold a lot of books.

After my accident, I somehow heard that the owner of this store had also been in an accident. It was many years earlier, but she suffered a head injury. The story was that her injury was part of the reason she started this spiritually based bookstore. She wanted work that mattered. One night in early spring, two years after my own book launch and about five months after my accident, there was a special event at her store for a Chicago psychic. My husband, Gary and I decided to go. Planning an outing like this was a big deal for us. Injury is a lonely state, especially with an injury that's unseen and difficult to describe. Still, I thought this event would give me a chance to get real, acknowledge my accident, and connect with understanding, safe and spiritual people.

Since the accident, I felt fragile and lost in groups of people. Gary was a great wingman that night, eventually maneuvering me through the crowd toward the owner. I wanted to connect with her. When the time seemed right, I pushed myself toward her and stuck out my hand.

"I'm Diane Wilson. You hosted my book launch a couple years ago."

"Yes, I remember. Good to see you!"

"Yes, I've been out. I had an accident and head injury." I thought this would make a connection.

Without any pause, she said, "I LOVE your shoes!"

Okay, my shoes were pretty cute. I had gotten them at Lori's on Armitage, and Lori has the world's best taste in stocking that store.

But I was stunned. This was my big venture out, and in trying to get real about my injury, this is what we were talking about?

I paused, unsure of how to respond.

"And I LOVE your hair! It's different, right?"

"Yes." A nod, then a handshake. It was the kind of handshake you know means "keep moving" even though she was smiling and warm.

"Great to see you. As always, thanks for such a great event," I said.

I stepped away and tried to blend back into the crowd.

Looking back, I am not sure what I was expecting was realistic—to bond around our injuries in her busy store during an event. And, if she also had a head injury, well, it wasn't fair of me to assume she would talk about it on demand. Further, she may have been struggling with her own cognitive and/or emotional limitations of being in a crowd, processing lots of different kinds of important information, remembering people and their stories, being social, and also managing the activities of a program she was sponsoring that night.

But at the time, it felt like: Here I am. It's such a big deal even to be here and say this, and you're talking about my SHOES, my HAIR!

This is reality for people with injuries or challenges on the inside, whether head injury, disease, or mental illness. If you look fine to others on the outside, you should be fine. It's how we are acculturated to digest that kind of information. Those assumptions and biases hurt the "invisible" wounded because it also makes it harder to listen to yourself, take yourself seriously, and seek the help you need.

Coffee with a Kind Friend

As I tested the edges of the small-plate universe I had created, I wanted to reconnect with some friends. One was from the Toastmasters group, where I had once been a member.

As a shy person, to prepare for the book launch in June 2004, I had taken months and months of training on how to give presentations without looking perfectly panicked. The Windy City Professional Speakers Toastmasters Club was my main prep group, where we videotaped our speeches and critiqued each other. This was innovative then, and only an especially brave or desperate contingent was attracted to this format. I had made lots of good friends in the group—doctors, salespeople, CEOs, small business owners, and lots of authors. I loved the group because major bonding occurs when confronting a primitive fear together, i.e., public speaking.

Six months after the accident, I had coffee with a friend from that group, and she just happened to be a neuropsychologist—Dr. Georgia Andrianopoulos. We sat in a small café near where our group had met in Oak Brook. She's Greek, strikingly beautiful with long blonde hair, and always clad in fashionable super-stylish clothes. Smart, kind, and truthful. As we caught up, I told her how happy I was to be almost finished dealing with the insurance company of the man whose car had hit me. I had finished PT in late March and was looking forward to settling the accident claim. That was my current story and understanding of my life, and where I'd been, though inside, I still felt fairly lost.

Georgia leaned over, looked me in the eyes kindly, raised one eyebrow ever so slightly, and said, "Dear, maybe you should have a brain scan before you settle... just in case." She could see what I could not.

Chapter 5:

What I Could Not See

Playing It Safe

Thinking I couldn't go wrong by playing it safe, I researched how to get a QEEG (quantitative electroencephalogram) brain scan, as my friend Georgia had recommended. Yes, it was prudent to get a completely clean bill of brain health before I settled my insurance claim.

My Internet research led me to psychologist Dr. Elsa Baehr. She was affiliated with Northwestern University, did some important research on depression, and was in private practice in Skokie, a suburb north of Chicago. She was considered a pioneer in the field of neurofeedback. Georgia approved of my choice.

Meeting Dr. Baehr was a turning point in my life in many ways, personally and professionally. A diminutive, elegant-looking clinician in a blue lab coat with dark, curly hair, she arranged for my testing with her staff and then interpreted the report. She was a true scientist and insisted on precisely collecting and explaining the data in ways I could understand. Just as important, she listened to me with her large, kind eyes and her heart. She was compassionate yet told the truth and could see the whole picture of me that I could not. Little by little, she guided me down a path that allowed me to identify and believe in my strengths and see my life in bigger ways. Over time, she provided the impetus to move forward in life and continues to do so. From the time I first met Dr. Baehr, I knew I wanted to be like her. I still do.

The QEEG Results

Dr. Baehr's desk was full of papers covered with little colored spheres representing my brain scan results. We went through them one by one.

She said my scan exhibited signature patterns of traumatic brain injury. She explained that with whiplash and concussion injuries, it's common for the front and back parts of the brain to no longer connect or communicate with each other optimally. The long nerve cells got stretched from the sudden snap forward of my head when my car was hit. Another related pattern was brainwave dysregulation around the front of my head. The image of dysregulated brain waves was shaped like a horseshoe with slower (delta and theta) waves dominating the forehead area—the prefrontal cortex—ending with the temples. The front houses the executive functions—planning, decision-making, and focus. My inner supervisor wasn't at her best, hence my dreamy, scattered, and dazed sense about things unless I was obsessing or hyper-focusing.

According to Dr. Baehr, the hyper-focus I experienced was a vestige of my attention deficit disorder. Ever since I was a young girl, if I was interested in something, I could focus for hours without a break. My husband would tell our friends about when I was writing Back in Control in our neighborhood Caribou coffee shop: he would visit me and then come back hours later, and I'd be in the same position still writing. An index measuring how likely it was that I had a moderate concussion registered 96%. That was a full seven months after the accident and after completing five months of physical therapy for my head and neck.

Despite the extent of my brain injury, my accident wasn't among the worst. It makes me wonder about the ones that are. I feel lucky to have found the path for recovery that I did.

Diagnosis

Nevertheless, I was surprised and sad that I was still injured and had spent so much time injured. After the accident, I had regularly seen very reputable physicians and other health care professionals from major Chicago health care systems. No one seemed to connect my dizziness, emotional roller coasters, and trouble focusing with something greater. Before the accident, I had written a book, been on TV and radio, and done countless book signings. After the October 2005 accident, my life was very different, and I had trouble keeping track of my wallet.

The diagnosis of traumatic brain injury still seven months after my accident was also a relief. It made sense out of many things, like why my life was not coming back together, even months after the accident. I found myself uncomfortable driving, and I could only take on tasks without much complexity. My confidence was low, my emotional life was consuming, and if I tried to pinpoint the issue, I just didn't feel strong or solid inside. Finally knowing the truth about my brain gave me hope, even though I was devastated and even embarrassed to realize I was that seriously injured. Dr. Baehr, or Elsa, as I came to call her, suggested she would treat me with neurofeedback to get my brain back in shape. Her recommendation gave me hope.

How Did I Not Know?

You may wonder how, months after my car accident, I did not know or realize I had a brain injury. [Footnote: Technically, concussion is, by definition, mild traumatic brain injury. What I had was a post-concussive disorder, a term not well-used at the time.] I have wondered so much about this myself. Putting together and writing my story has helped me understand this better. It's still stunning to me, though, how this phase of my life was and how lucky I was to find help to move forward. I hope others who hear my story will become more aware of these shadowy symptoms, make the connections of their symptoms to their injury more quickly, and seek help with persistence. I also hope they find the resources they need to heal. These are all my hopes.

First, even though I saw well-intended health care professionals, no one seemed to notice my brain injury or labeled it to me as such. The word concussion was used at first, but after months, I was treated particularly in physical therapy for whiplash. Other than my husband, I'm not sure others appreciated what had happened to my brain. Perhaps, because the physical therapist had not known me before the accident, she didn't recognize how much less present and less focused I was and how I was functioning at a much lower level in every element of my life.

Before the accident, I had a full-time private practice in downtown Chicago, seeing very successful clients who were fine-tuning their work behavior and planning their next career steps. I had been promoting my book. Just prior to that, I was a regular contributor to a column in the *Chicago Tribune*, which put my face on the cover page of the Sunday newspaper distributed to 2.5 million homes. Fast forward to doing months of physical therapy and being stuck to a screen, trading stocks in the bedroom of my condo.

When I learned Dr. Baehr's diagnosis, I talked to Dr. Locke. She said concussions can take a while to heal. Although she supported every treatment option suggested to me—like months of physical therapy and acupuncture, perhaps she expected my brain would get better on its own over time. Perhaps in my dealings with all my other caregivers, there was a perceptual bias: I looked healthy and put together. Maybe it's harder to digest the possibility of an injury or deficit, or maybe people assumed this was just the new me. I'm sure there are things about this I will never understand.

What about the psychotherapist/psychiatrist I'd seen once a month for many years? He didn't help me understand what was going on with me. Why didn't he provide more help with medical referrals or information? He's never been one to answer a lot of questions. Instead, he deflected things back with the question, "How do you feel about that?"

Yes, he has a beard like Freud. I was angry when I learned the diagnosis and stopped seeing him for a time. I felt he wasn't doing his job—either he didn't see my struggles (impossible to believe) or wasn't honest with me. I wonder if he didn't have any ideas on how to help me either—no one did. How horrifying it would be to see someone you've known so long, place her injured life in front of you once a month. Certainly, he has limitations, yet I do know he cared, tried to observe me in the best way he could, and had been a steady rock in the stormier parts of my life. After five months, I started seeing him again. I recently told him he needs to read Chapter Three of this book very carefully.

My husband loves me unconditionally and was worried, but I think he was just glad that I was alive. Events like this teach us that life can change rather quickly. Yet, I know he also felt helpless, like we were doing the best we could with the situation. He didn't know what else he or anyone could do.

Perhaps the most important question about this diagnosis is: How did I keep my brain injury from myself?

Remember the GPS I discussed in Chapter Two? The brain can keep redirecting itself without yelling that you made a bad turn—a seamless process of unconsciously redirecting. In my case, the GPS bypassed awareness of my mental and psychological limitations. It didn't contribute to an update of my identity—"This is me now after this accident. This is how I am." Instead, I didn't feel or recognize my cognitive limitations at the time. The frontal lobes of my brain, where self-awareness and identity are largely housed, were impaired.

In writing this manuscript, editors have asked me repeatedly how I reacted to the losses I experienced during this time. I didn't recognize the losses as such. I didn't even see them or use other executive functions of planning, looking ahead, figuring out what I needed to do to create a future because my focus, like that of most sick people, was on the present, getting through the week. It's like when we visit someone in a hospital. We wouldn't dream of talking about the weather because it's not part of the patient's focus. Instead, the patient is focused on eating, drinking, going to the bathroom—all more immediate needs.

Especially at first, I didn't suffer the months when I wasn't contributing to my retirement funds. After a few months, I developed an obsessive focus—it is common for those with brain injury to have obsessive thinking. It was for trading those funds in the stock market: something I could watch and see in that very moment.

My self-awareness gaps showed with the food bank Green Shirt team, not appreciating that I was team-building with a team that I really wasn't on. And I was very happy doing it, even if the team's manager wasn't. The phobic behavior in the car, screaming out directions to my husband since I thought cars were coming at us. There was an awareness in the moment that this wasn't right but also an inability to observe my behaviors within a bigger picture. Over and over, it didn't happen.

I tell the Green Shirt story now and understand how my lack of awareness was related to my injury, but it was years before I could understand what had happened that day. Instead, the scene was logged with a question mark in my mind; I knew there was something important about the frustrated manager saying, "Only green shirts in the picture." I had just been glad to be somewhere working with people, using my body and brain. If you want to know what it feels like for some of us who have had an injury with something as basic as our brain, this is what it can be like. These symptoms are hard to imagine unless it's happened to you.

Originally, I was diagnosed with having a moderate concussion. After seven months, I had what's called "post-concussion syndrome," which is, according to the Mayo Clinic:

"... a complex disorder in which various symptoms—such as headaches and dizziness—last for weeks and sometimes months after the injury that caused the concussion."[2]

Post-concussion syndrome helped explain some things to me,

2 https://www.mayoclinic.org/diseases-conditions/post-concussion-syndrome/symptoms-causes/syc-20353352

like why my capacity was limited and why I didn't feel like going to professional meetings or taking on new projects, but moment to moment, I could rarely hold the thought or insight that I had brain trauma. I always felt like I was a pretty smart person since I did well in school. I felt I was doing okay.

I've mentioned the moment of understanding I had shortly after the accident when I was able to understand my childhood neighbor who was developmentally disabled in a new way. But that understanding of myself and my own brain dissipated quickly. I didn't identify personally with being injured after that initial insight. In about 2011, I wrote about concussion in a couple of articles for our town paper, one on the movie *Concussion*. I disclosed that I had recovered from a traumatic brain injury, but I didn't grasp the reality of what that meant. I still wasn't making the connection between this injury and its impact on my life and the kinds of damage the football players I was writing about had. Part of that may have been because massive damage is easier to understand than the more subtle changes of personality, focus, and emotions.

It's hard to convey this lack of self-awareness. Oliver Sacks discusses it in his book *The Man Who Mistook His Wife for a Hat*.

Here's another example: about eight months after the accident, I ran into an attorney, Antonio, who had shared a downtown office near mine a couple of years before. I saw him after I had taken some time off and come back to my practice. He knew people in the suite I shared with him. We passed each other on the sidewalk in front of the beautiful gothic Fourth Presbyterian church on Michigan Avenue. I always liked Antonio and was genuinely happy to see him. A kind man, he stopped and looked into my eyes with concern and said: "How ARE you?"

I was totally surprised and said: "Fine. Things are okay." I had no idea why he was looking at me so intently with concern. My having been injured was totally off my radar. I didn't connect with that part of our short conversation until later when I told my husband about the exchange. We figured it out. Now, I am certain he knew about my accident and injury even though he wouldn't say that. I felt bad about it; he was so nice, and I was so clueless. Most people didn't ask me about it, and I certainly had no way yet to talk about it.

Here's another factor: Yes, I didn't identify with the question of an injury-related illness, but even if I had, could you imagine any potential room in a conversation for an exchange like, "Yes, my brain is still pretty foggy, I get dizzy, and my obsessive focus is much worse, but I'm coming back." Could you imagine an honest conversation on any level with most other people about such an injury? I love people in general, but I believe many don't care to hear about brain health issues. I am hoping they will want to read about them, though.

For me, all signs reinforced my own internal process of "Ignore this injury, and it will go away." That's another reason why I'm writing this book—to help provide a framework for dialogue about such a vexing injury. It's also to warn you that if your spouse, friend, or child has a head injury and goes to see a doctor, you may do well to go with them to provide a bigger picture for the healthcare professional in case your loved one can't. Because if they are like me, they won't report what a spouse or close friend could observe. My spouse was so supportive in me getting whatever help I needed. An advocate of the truest stripe. But I could not imagine him seeing my doctor by himself saying: "When will I get my wife back?" It was too unreal, too painful. I think Gary thought we were doing the best we could in my healing, and he hoped I would just get better. He never bargained for this, and my heart aches thinking about what he went through.

My awareness and language for talking about the post-concussion symptoms were limited. I knew it made an impact to say I had a head injury, but I had no idea how to integrate awareness of its impact on my own life or keep in mind that this described me. I remember telling a super smart and accomplished friend early in February 2006 about the concussion, just after reading her beautiful annual Christmas card. She said:

"How does it affect you?"

Pause.

"Does it make things like organization and focus harder?"

These seemed like great questions but not ones I could answer very well. I recall agreeing that it made organizing and focus harder, but the correct answer was that the part of me that could evaluate my skills was also affected. If I talked about those deficits, it would mean that I could separate them from the rest of me, that I had a self I was aware of. But my self-awareness and my self-knowledge were exactly the parts of me impaired by the injury.

Getting back to Chapter One: On the list of concussion symptoms, I believe it would be valuable to add the symptom of impaired self-awareness. Of course, you can see how complicated this could be from a legal perspective in terms of treatment—do you treat someone who doesn't know they need it? Make them take medicine? Do we let them play football when they are not the ones who can decide what's best if they are injured? These are vexing questions.

Anosognosia

The medical term for this aspect of my injury is called anosognosia. It means a lack of insight or awareness. The term was coined in 1892 by the early neurologist Joseph Babinski in 1914. "Anosognosia" comes from the Greek word for disease (*nosos*) and knowledge (*gnosis*). It literally means "to not know a disease." (source: ask)[3]

Anosognosia affects 50% of people with schizophrenia and 40% with bipolar illness and is the single most significant reason these patients don't want to take their medicine.[4] Lack of insight and awareness is not the same as denial. It is likely based on an injury, and research hypothesizes that different locations of the brain could be the source. More recent summaries of the literature point to the impaired connections between various brain areas— particularly the communications with the frontal, side (temporal),

---

3   https://en.wikipedia.org/wiki/Anosognosia
4   https://www.treatmentadvocacycenter.org/key-issues/anosognosia

and back right (parietal) parts of the brain. It is common in strokes and different types of brain injury, yet it is something I have rarely seen discussed in relation to concussion. As someone who had a concussion where I couldn't see my injury that clearly, I certainly wish someone would have mentioned this or that I could have read about it.

With anosognosia, awareness is relative, and a person can be aware at one point and not at others. My awareness felt like Swiss cheese. At times, I could grasp that I wasn't the same old me, but in terms of keeping that in mind in dealing with others, it didn't happen. I couldn't digest that I was injured, or if I did, my awareness came and went. I couldn't see my injury very well or think about it realistically until I was far along in my healing. I didn't feel grief for what I had lost because I often was unaware of what was gone. I wrestled with a range of feelings. It's like I was aware of something that was missing but couldn't put my words together to describe it. It was a very strange experience.

The Injured Self

In terms of my sense of self, the prefrontal cortex shapes our experience of ourselves, self-awareness. When all goes well, it reshapes as we change. Example: If we learn a new skill, we incorporate it into our identity/sense of being and see ourselves as someone who can do X (the new skill). When this part of the brain is injured or compromised, as with bipolar illness, brain injury, and dementia, self-awareness isn't updated. It's like the elderly parent who no longer has the skills to drive but can't see or retain that awareness. They haven't updated their sense of self to digest it.

This is undoubtedly a major factor in why people with injuries don't seek help, keep playing football, or refuse to take their medication when it's critical. They can't see or remember that they are compromised. Can an injured sports player really decide whether they are impaired?

In coaching, psychotherapy, and any kind of personal transformation process, the awareness of self and behavior is fundamental and yet, in some cases, cannot be taken for granted.

The Next Turn

Getting back to my QEEG results and Elsa's recommendation to start neurofeedback: no one else had a better idea or, for that matter, any idea of what I should do next. There was nothing on the horizon for improving my life as I stood with my gold star in PT behind me. So, I was in. Besides, learning about the brain had long been a passion, and you know me and mother figures like my teachers and Dr. Locke. I loved Elsa from the moment I met her. To be fair, everyone loves Elsa. However, I felt she could understand me in ways I couldn't and would help me change my life.

Chapter 6:

Levying the Costs

Four Trains and a Taxi

By the time I started sessions with Elsa in May 2006, I was driving our car. Because my appointments were during the week and my husband and I then shared a car, I commuted via public transportation from our home in suburban Oak Park to her office in Skokie on Chicago's North Shore. My husband picked me up in Skokie after my appointment, and he got out of work in Elk Grove Village. For those unfamiliar with Chicagoland, just know the distance traveled for me and my husband was significant. Then there was the convenience factor. My path to get to my session: I walked from our condo, through Scoville Park to the commuter train platform (seven minutes), caught the Chicago Transit Authority (CTA) Green Line to downtown Chicago (thirty minutes), took the Brown Line north to its end at the Howard Station (forty minutes), got on the Purple Line to the Yellow Line (another forty minutes), and went to the end of the Yellow Line in Skokie (ten minutes). Finally, I hopped in a cab for a two-mile ride to her office. $4.50 plus tip. How had I decided that neurofeedback was something to commit to doing when it entailed all that and a forty-five-minute trip home in the car?

Many Beautiful Threads

Like the back of a hand-woven rug, there were many threads woven into my belief that doing neurofeedback with Elsa was the right thing for me. I described my response to her personally, liking her very much from the beginning. But even before learning about neurofeedback, I sensed things that I would later recognize were much more relevant than I had realized at the time. Most important, sometimes my barriers, the blocks, felt like "a brain thing." That was an expression people used during that time—it's a brain thing—and I did too. It shows how deeply intuitive we can be about our illness and bodies—even if that wisdom doesn't reach our conscious awareness. It was an expression that fit when you forgot your keys or hesitated in finding the word you wanted to say. But this was an insight that sat in my deepest consciousness like a repeating shape or image you might see in your mind's eye during your sleep. It had a trueness that doesn't connect with anything real or concrete. You just knew it was there. That's as much as my mind would let me know.

When I was growing up, my dad was a self-taught electronics buff—meaning he sent away for Heath kits and made things like televisions in the basement in the evenings. We lived in the country, and one year, he taught a 4-H program on electronics. I clearly recall the little snippets of wires and cables he had all arranged and stapled down, side by side on a piece of hardwood board for the group. In his soft, unassuming manner and deep fascination with learning, he explained what the wires were made of and how each was different. I remember nothing about the specifics of electrical wires. Instead, my prize was being imprinted with the belief that I didn't need to be afraid of technical things. My dad's 4-H program didn't just demystify things technical; it made them all the more fascinating. I acquired a confidence that technical activities could be part of my world too. Certainly, much has changed since my 4-H club and Dad's Heath kits. But, I learned neurofeedback involved placing electrical sensor wires on the head. I was intrigued instead of intimidated. No problem.

Since college, prior to the Decade of the Brain, designated in 1990 by the first President Bush, I had been drawn to anything "brain." In studying clinical and counseling psychology for my master's degree, I loved the physiological psychology classes and struggled with losing that focus as I made career and organizational development my specialty. As a graduate student at the University of Akron in Ohio, I had some part-time work in the practice of one of my professors, giving assessments to brain-injured patients working for the department of vocational resources. I loved it. But post-injury, these experiences felt like a different lifetime and had dropped out of my awareness completely.

My natural tendencies, though, persisted and popped out in humorous ways. Example: Just before my accident, I remember having some friends stay over and carefully preparing our bedroom to be their sleeping space. I looked around the sky-colored room with the large brown, wooden headboard, fresh sheets, and collection of large comfy pillows. My eye caught the nightstand anew. I realized I needed to deconstruct my sleep comfort zone for our guests. Next to my pillow was a stack of four to six brain books I loved to read at night. These included Daniel Amen's books on ADD, *Change Your Brain, Change Your Life,* and more. Like many people with ADD, I enjoy reading more than one book at a time. I realized all the brain books might seem a little strange. Even now, my relatives tease me that I am the only person they know who reads neuroscience texts and *People* magazine before I go to sleep. Brain science was my private passion. I studied. In retrospect, I knew next to nothing about the brain or how it worked. Still, I loved it.

Another thread came from when I was investigating neurofeedback before meeting with Elsa. I came across a study that showed that children with ADD who were trained with neurofeedback had an average gain of sixteen points on IQ tests. While my therapist's perspective is that neurofeedback was "on the fringe," away from traditional medicine, traditional medicine had yet to offer me much vis-à-vis my own brain injury: nothing much except a "wait and see" attitude to find my way back to a normal life. He said he thought it couldn't hurt. Dr. Locke was very open to new cutting-edge approaches. After clearing it with them both, I felt intrigued and excited to start neurofeedback.

I had neurofeedback treatments once or twice a week for over two years, from April 2006 to June 2008. It was an unusual and valuable phase of my life. I'll talk more about what neurofeedback is and how my treatment progressed in the next chapter, But here, I'll tell you about what the process and commitment entailed. If not threads of a hand-woven rug, you see the stones hidden just under the water lined up to make my path into this treatment and my recovery a natural one. However, it was one that was not without a significant personal cost.

My Train Rides with Eckhart

Almost two years prior, in June 2003, I had attended Book Expo in New York City, which is a large international book conference where publishers generously share key releases from their lineups. It's a big book giveaway with people carrying home huge bags of new books. Wandering through the aisles of booths, I met a representative from a relatively small company called New World Library who said they had an exceptional book that season from an author named Eckhart Tolle called *Stillness Speaks*. They gave me a free advanced copy. Along with *The Power of Now*, it would become one of the most important books of the time, maybe of all times, on spiritual guidance. Tolle's beautiful writings are a guide to find the power of being in the moment, to empty the mind of the nagging, negative chatter that can torture us endlessly. He teaches us how to find the stillness that lies beneath the internal noise.

His books and audios were a huge comfort in the phase of my life following the accident. I read the books, underlined and revisited key phrases, and even had purchased flashcards of the inspiring quotes. Here are two of my favorites:

Whenever you notice that some form of negativity has arisen within you, look on it not as a failure, but as a helpful signal that is telling you:

Wake up. Get out of your mind. Be present. You can always cope with the now, but you can never cope with the future—nor do you have to. The answer, the strength, the right action, or the resource will be there when you need it, not before, not after. From the book *The Power of Now.* Copyright © 2004 by Eckhart Tolle. Reprinted with Permission by New World Library, Novato, CA. www.newworldlibrary.com.

I put his CDs in my Sony Walkman and listened to them daily—before going to sleep, on the train, anywhere. Like one of Pavlov's dogs, to this day, all I have to do is hear Tolle's voice to instantly breathe in and bring my mind to my breath. His funny laugh always makes me laugh.

There were many good days during this time. Life was a teacher, and on a good day, I could feel the bliss of the moment. I realized that I am a body, mind, and a spiritual being in this life. My path was not everyone's. I could see that since I didn't keep regular hours in regular places, spent a fair amount of time taking care of my body—exercise and acupuncture—and, full-disclosure, continued my hobby of researching and trading stocks. Tolle's books offered spiritual guidance that augmented the progress I was making through neurofeedback. I was practicing being present, taking nothing for granted, a person whose life was under construction. His guidance was a salve to help me in the treatment itself but also in my life, to not think very far ahead and to appreciate the present. Life wasn't perfect, but it was my teacher, and so was Eckhart Tolle. Thank you, Eckhart.

About TKD

After my break in late 2005, I returned to TKD and had continued as consistently as I could. The TKD club was a part of my exercise plan and my social life and had been for six years. Learning a contact sport together with others is bonding. Before the accident, I sometimes spent time practicing with other members and celebrating birthdays and holidays at occasional parties. Over the years, one generous member had made the first and most beautiful website for my company. Another was a lawyer who provided me with insight before signing a leasing agreement my company needed. Members were interesting, from all different paths. One guy who was involved in the club for a while had been an Illinois State Senator, then a U.S. Senator, and finally, the forty-fourth president of the United States. Yep, Barack Obama. It was an interesting and exciting connection.

But after I returned from my break in late 2005, I would periodically get injured in class. It rarely happened before the accident that I recall. Now it happened about every two or three weeks. Everyone knew I had had a head injury and couldn't take direct hits. Still, somehow, I'd get hit. For example, my teacher, who knew my situation, somehow ended up hitting me in the process of demonstrating moves, punches, or whatever. A hard punch to my body would reverberate into my head. Even wearing protective gear, I could feel the impact. It seemed like I should be able to take it in stride—and I wanted to—but I would feel dizzy and queasy and not like myself for at least a day afterward. I loved my TKD club, but somehow the injuries kept happening.

I loved what TKD required from me: physical skill, perceptiveness of others, movement, and stamina. Maybe there were students better and learned faster than me, but no one loved it more. Being a martial artist was part of who I was, my identity. No one seemed to understand the cost I was paying through these cycles of injury and recovery. I didn't share much about how it affected me when I saw stars from an accidental hit or someone bumping into me. No one could help me evaluate if continuing TKD was right for me at that time.

Until Elsa.

Shortly after I started my treatment with her, I came into my appointment feeling the effects of class the night before and mentioned it. I learned fast that you might as well tell Elsa the things you don't want her to know since somehow, someway, she would know any way, or you'd be there spilling the beans on her terms. She asked about everything—how I was sleeping, what I did with my time, was I doing my homework, sex—everything. Also, this kind, smart, and perceptive clinician had a way of looking right through you even if you weren't talking.

Our conversation that day happened while she was placing sensors on my head for the training. She bent down and situated herself—black mascara, long eyelashes, crinkly eyes, red lipstick, this tiny frame in her blue lab coat—to be at eye-level with me. At five feet, nine inches tall, even sitting in the treatment chair, I was almost the same size as Elsa was standing up. Still, it happened like this:

"Diane, if you are hurt or have been hurt in your TKD class, you need to stop going. Your brain can't heal if you keep re-injuring it."

There, she'd said it. That was a relief. That seemed hard to hear but somehow fair. My brain was getting reinjured when I took a hit. Still, I was basking in her attention and felt there was probably a little wiggle-room on the whole decision of whether to participate in TKD. She was such a kind and diplomatic person; she understood that I loved the sport. Elsa liked me and thought it was interesting that I had this exotic skill in martial arts, breaking boards and all. She wanted me to be happy.

It soon became clear I was reading this all wrong.

"If you don't quit, I can't work with you anymore."

Wow, just like that! You'd abandon me for that? What will happen to me, my life, and all the good things you said my treatment could bring—feeling better, more focused, and having a full life?

Surprised, it took a minute, but then I got it. This wasn't a topic for negotiation. And if I wanted to be onboard for working with her to change my life, I needed to fall into line. There would be no TKD martial arts or anything where I could re-injure my head. She wasn't putting time into saving my brain so someone in my TKD club could swing carelessly and turn me into pudding. She was unwilling to ignore what I wanted to wallpaper over—I was allowing myself to be in a situation where I could be injured, however it happened. There was a resolute dignity she had about her time, her work, and, most importantly, my future.

But I needed to take a big step I hadn't anticipated and wasn't ready to take.

Losing My Art, Losing Myself

I stumbled out of Elsa's office that day, told my husband what happened, and then made the decision to quit TKD. It was over. I felt bare. Of all the things that happened during the seven months after the accident, this was the hardest. Many things I could ignore, mute, or overlook. This wasn't one of them. For six years before my accident, I'd spent at least two, and often three, days a week in TKD class. Between classes, I often did workouts for conditioning for strength and flexibility and practiced my TKD forms. My life was, in part, defined and grounded by martial arts training. It anchored me. But I wanted to work with Elsa.

I searched for something to replace TKD. It was a dull gap in my life that I never knew how I'd fill. Some women with lockers near mine at my club said they loved water aerobics. Loved, loved, loved it. I only went once: the one-piece bathing suits, the tight bathing cap that hurt my head, silver-haired women wearing lipstick and big bangles and necklaces, all of us bobbing to Broadway show tunes in the chilly water. It wasn't for me. I loved those ladies, but it wasn't my sport. I missed being strong, fighting with the boys and winning, and all the thrill and challenges of TKD.

It felt impossible to continue to be a member of that health club without belonging to TKD. So, I quit and joined a gym closer to my home. No Barack Obama and family. No other things and people as cool as at the gym downtown. But then, I wasn't that cool anymore either. The loss was a significant one, disorienting on a daily basis, but I somehow sealed that over in my mind and wouldn't let myself dwell on it.

So much in my life had changed. I rarely looked to the future and took nothing for granted. This wasn't completely bad. I made daily gratitude lists of all the things I had, like a wonderful husband and a nice home where I felt safe. Daily I watched Oprah (but no TV after her eleven a.m. show) and embraced the age-old wisdom of what Buddhists call "impermanence," meaning nothing lasts forever—either good or bad. Also, prominent in my mind remained that whatever your circumstance, nothing was guaranteed. I tried to stay in the moment like a little snail in its shell.

Chapter 7:

The Brain Training Begins!

The Magic?

Each of the sessions with Dr. Baehr was designed like this: first, a brief one-on-one conversation with Elsa to check in on how I was doing—feeling, thinking, and what I was doing between sessions—and then I worked with her and/or her interns on neurofeedback and a range of other applied neuroscience tools to heal and rewire my brain.

At my very first training session, Elsa had said she wanted to show me this exciting technique. It was very powerful, and I could even do it at home.

"Great, what is it?

"It's breathing," she said deliberately and then smiled.

"Oh..." I already knew how to breathe. *What did I sign-up for here?!*

Heart Rate Variability (HRV)

Elsa pinched open a clip and attached it to my ear. I love electrical gadgets and was liking the idea better already. She explained this was a biofeedback device that would measure the variability of my heart rate. Biofeedback entails you getting information or feedback about the state or activity of a body system. In this case, it was my heart. HRV describes the range from maximum heart rate (which occurs during the inhale) to your minimum (during the exhale). This reflects the balance of the autonomic nervous system. It's an important concept in health and healing: smoother, deeper breathing patterns are much better. So, the variability of the heart rate (meaning differences in pattern) is ideally high. This is best achieved through abdominal breathing. Or so I learned.

Elsa then played a vocal coaching DVD from Stephen Elliott, who was a friend of hers. Even at that early point, I could gather that Dr. Baehr knew almost everyone, and everyone was happy to be her friend.

In his deep, resonant voice, Stephen counted, "INHALE 2-3-4 EXHALE 2-3-4," over and over and over. This particular count is for what he calls "coherent breathing." He has written a great deal about this pattern of rhythmicity and depth considered optimal for brain-body balance.

The challenge was to breathe to the count through my abdomen... my belly. No matter how hard I tried, my belly would stay super still, and my chest would look like I just ran a race. I tried putting one hand on my chest and the other on the belly. Nope. The harder I tried, the more my chest heaved up and down. I wasn't very good at this.

During the treatment, with a device on my ear, I watched my heart rate activity on a screen. When breathing patterns were consistent (all heartbeat tracings looping smoothly across the screen), I heard that pleasant tone. If my breathing became less rhythmic, the pleasant tones stopped.

I was relieved to notice I wasn't the only patient in the clinic who struggled with what should be a simple act. Some patients, however, appeared to be champs right from the beginning. I would see them with their therapist filing into one of the small treatment rooms, and within seconds, I could hear the sound that signaled they were doing better than I was. It's not that I cared much about listening and comparing myself to other people in the clinic or that doing well there wasn't the biggest thing I had going on in my life. Nope, none of that. But, of course, the opposite was true.

Vagus the "Wandering" Nerve

Abdominal breathing is v-e-r-y important for the body. It helps orchestrate a rhythm that affects everything by stimulating the vagus nerve. That's the only one of the twelve cranial nerves that goes outside the skull. It's anchored in the spinal cord and brain stem, and, as the longest cranial nerve, it wanders through the body, touching almost every single organ. It interfaces with the parasympathetic (calming) nervous system, influencing our lungs, heart, and digestive system. Abdominal breathing tones the vagus nerve to calm our systems from a stress mode to more optimal daily functioning. It affects our gut, where 95% of the serotonin ("feel-good" neurotransmitter) for our brain is produced. It also hones our gut instincts. It allows the whole body to get in sync, balancing the nervous system, healing the body, teaching focus, and even potentially improving our golf and tennis games.

Since we've been breathing our whole lives, our breathing patterns are deeply embedded, unconscious habits. But breathing is also one of the few unconscious body activities where we can also exert conscious control. Because of its unconscious habitual role in daily life, the patterns can be very hard to change.

Once I learned how to breathe (that's how we'd say it, referring to abdominal breathing), we went on to the next steps. I used to joke that I had been breathing wrong and didn't even know it! While I had to learn to breathe to do my brain training, the heart rate variability (HRV) training WAS my brain training.

"Breathing" Homework

My homework from Elsa was to practice at least five minutes a day, preferably in the morning just after waking up (although doing it in the evening can help with sleep). Ultimately, a good goal is twenty minutes a day.

I had purchased the biofeedback device myself from Heartmath. com and loved using it at home, on the train, in the waiting room, or any place. The effect of rhythmic breathing for an extended period can be profound. It improves sleep, anxiety, mood, and focus. For me, everything. I experience life more fully when I do regular HRV training. It wasn't until my psychotherapist asked me a question about this that I crystalized what was happening.

"What does this breathing do for you?"

"Well... when I don't do the breathing session to start the day, I feel like a person who's sketched on paper with straight black lines. A stick person. When I do the breathing practice, I am colored in; I feel richer, fuller. I know how I feel about things. I'm more decisive and ready to act in a deliberate way."

Okay... Who could argue his goofy questions didn't help at points?

Not Everyone Should Meditate

Often it seems the recommendation is that everyone should meditate, that it's good for all of us. For people like me, it wasn't the next recommended step. I was too unfocused and emotionally fragile to sit still with my eyes closed and try not to pay attention to my mind. There was no meditation style I knew of where I could be comfortable when I started my treatment with Elsa. My time of guided listening to Eckhart's CDs and the practice of finding stillness were good. However, this HRV biofeedback device gave me a way of structuring a journey toward relaxation and creating a different brain state than I had otherwise. It was like finding the stairway and a handrail to bring me to the next level of the brain state— lower arousal and increased focus. I love it since the software creates graphs of overall progress and could show a chart of the day's activity. It gives very tangible feedback during the training and afterward.

Knowledge Versus Habit

Understanding the benefits of balancing the nervous system and creating relaxation and focus is one thing. But cultivating abdominal breathing as a habit didn't happen right away. I remember one day rushing into the clinic ten minutes late. It was late summer, and I was driving myself by then, and I had been snagged by a long freight train. I sat there panicked, drumming my nails on the steering wheel, until finally, the last train car passed, and I could be on my way to Elsa's office. I got there, and my heart rate was 115 beats per minute as I kept explaining what happened. Elsa interrupted me twice to say: *"What about the breathing?"* I thought she was scolding me since I was late and would not be doing the breathing when I should have been here in the office.

"No, I really couldn't get here since the train cars just kept coming!"

Finally, she rested her hand on my knee and said: "Diane, what I am saying is that the breathing is for stress, and you can practice it in your car as well as in the office. You can use this breathing practice whenever you're stressed."

Okay... I knew that. But I didn't know that. And certainly, I didn't know it at the habit level. Now, after years of training myself, if I'm stressed, I will inhale through my nose and feel my tummy (not lungs) expand. It always helps.

Back to my first session.

Finally, the Good Stuff—EEG-based Neurofeedback

The second part of the training was the EEG-based neurofeedback itself. I was psyched for this part. I asked Elsa about that study I came across that found neurofeedback could increase IQ by sixteen points. She knew of the research that involved children with ADD. She said it didn't surprise her since focus, concentration, mental flexibility, memory, information processing speed, and other cognitive skills can be enhanced by neurofeedback.

"Things will feel easier, even things that weren't hard," she told me.

Dr. Baehr was working with adults who were struggling in college or grad school, people who had had injuries like a stroke, cancer patients suffering fuzzy chemo brain, and treating resistant depression—people who had tried many treatments that didn't help. More than traditional intelligence, she also said it helped with emotional intelligence by increasing the ability to manage emotions and impulses, to listen to and read other people more realistically, and to handle stress without it impacting communications. That all sounded good to me. I was ready for phase two. But let's address some basics.

Origins of Neurofeedback

Neurofeedback is biofeedback for the brain. Biofeedback gives the body information about what it is doing (like a mirror), so it can adjust and be more effective. It involves rewarding the more optimal behaviors. That's like getting cash at the ATM when we push the right buttons. In neurofeedback, the brain gets information about the brain waves being produced and rewards those that are most optimal. If this doesn't make a lot of sense, no worries. It will as we go along.

The field was founded in the early 1920s by German psychiatrist Hans Berger, who is most well-known for discovering a method to record and monitor brain waves (electroencephalography, EEG) as well as the alpha wave, which is also referred to as the Berger Wave. Then in the mid-1960s, researcher Dr. Joe Kamiya at the University of Chicago discovered that he could teach his subjects to regulate their levels of alpha waves. These are the early roots of modern brain training.

Different Types of Brain Waves

In addition to the alpha wave, a spectrum of brain wave types has been identified. They are categorized in terms of Hertz, or cycles of energy waves per second, as well as, to some degree, their shape. Alpha waves have a frequency of loops of eight to twelve cycles per second. They are smooth loops, not jagged, and are associated with an internal focus and calmness. You may have heard people say that yoga increases their alpha waves, a feel-good experience. Here are the other main categories of brain waves based on their shape and frequency, too.

- Delta (very slow waves, 0.5-4 Hz, associated with injury and being deeply tired). Infants begin life with more slow waves than adults but this changes as we grow older and become more active. My injury was diagnosed in part by excess delta and theta in the frontal lobe. This makes sense because my head jolted forward upon impact, bouncing my brain to the front part of my skull, creating the injury.

- Theta (5-8 Hz, the brainwave of pre-consciousness, internal focus). If you stepped into the local Walgreen's drug store, totally forgetting why you went there and started to remember a dream you had last night, likely theta waves are dominant. One of the several types of ADD has the hallmark of too much theta and not enough beta, making an individual spacey and distracted and challenged in managing time and making decisions. With traumatic brain injury (TBI), it is not surprising to find too much theta in the executive function areas, too, such as I had, making it very hard to stay goal-centered or realistic about time and life. Theta will be increased by some types of meditation as it is considered a slow wave and also present during sleep.

- Alpha (8-12 Hz) as discussed above.

- Beta (12-30 Hz) is associated with an external focus versus being focused on your own internal experience, oriented to solve problems and act upon the environment versus procrastinate, such as when theta dominates in the executive function.

- High Beta (30-40 Hz) is a very fast brain wave, like a "pedal to the metal" state. It's associated with rumination, irritability. It's sometimes considered a high peak performance state and is also thought more recently to reflect muscular tension—the electric potential generated by muscle cells when activated, for example, from tension in the back of the head and neck.

There is much more to all this, but this basic information provides a start. Each brain wave contributes to different mental states. Ideally, the brain can produce all these different wavebands that operate in the same way as when driving a car. You want to be able to go slow and fast as the situation requires and also move flexibly (not get stuck on one speed). When Kamiya trained an individual to produce alpha waves, the world of brain science should have been turned on its ear. If you can teach a person to change the brain, it moves us toward realizing we are not these permanently fixed creations that only grow older and decline. We can control and change our brain—that's neuroplasticity, a whole new paradigm of thinking. However, few people had heard about it or appreciated its worth at the time, and neurofeedback is still a well-kept secret compared to innovations in the pharmaceutical industry where the funding for product marketing is vastly different.

The largest amount of research has been done with ADHD (attention deficit hyperactivity disorder), where there is compelling evidence that neurofeedback can make significant and long-lasting improvements. Neurofeedback is also used for anxiety, depression, learning disabilities, and more. Professional athletes, several high-profile Olympians, and Olympic teams rely on neurofeedback to give a competitive advantage by increasing mental focus and resilience. It is more popular in Europe than the United States.

As the technology develops, we are likely to see more of neurofeedback. For example, having an fMRI (functional magnetic resonance imaging) makes the training activity easier to monitor more precisely.

You Want Me to What?!

To begin, Elsa's assistant, Kim, put sensors on my head. These are not called electrodes due to the negative baggage of that term, as in electrocution. Also, they really do only "sense"—listen to and monitor—brain waves, not deliver any type of electrical charge. First, she rubbed my scalp at predetermined spots with an aqua-colored, mildly abrasive gel to exfoliate the surface. It wasn't painful, although she did rub these spots pretty hard. She said this exfoliation improves the sensor's ability to connect and listen to the electrical activity beneath it. She scooped an electro-conductive paste into tiny, golden cups at the end of the sensors and pressed each onto my scalp. She strategically targeted areas that the scan showed brain wave activity that was too high, too low, disconnected, or unequal. Overall, no matter how lovely my hair looked before the session, it stuck close to my head afterward. Totally worth it.

After Elsa checked for sensor location and connection, the neurofeedback training began.

"See this thermometer on the screen?" Elsa said.

"Yes?" A single blue thermometer bobbed away, up and down. High, then low.

"Keep it under this line." It was busy hovering well above the line.

"Er... how?"

"You'll learn."

No joystick. No levers. Just my brain. Okay...

I shook my head and squinted my eyes. *No go.*

"Okay, adjust my brain waves? But how?"

"Just breathe."

Oh yeah, that... okay?

"And observe what you're doing or feeling when the thermometer comes down and try to do or feel more of that."

The first few sessions were the hardest. I had simply no idea what was going on or how to control my brain waves. The technical goal of this first training exercise was to reduce the amplitude of theta at CZ. Elsa said most people do not feel they have any control over their brain waves during the first four to six sessions. I was worried because it was clear I absolutely had no idea how to make the bouncing thermometer go higher or lower or do anything at all. She reasserted that no one could possibly know how to do any of this, and if she explained too much, it could get in the way of me finding the gear levers within myself.

I'd stare at the bouncing blue thermometer and try to relax and focus as instructed. On the focus part, it was hard to figure out how to make my brain do this or even what it meant. Sometimes my eyes would feel like they were bugging out as I stared at the screen, trying harder and harder. That didn't help at all, and Elsa said I was trying too hard. Finally, one of the interns suggested being like a cat, relaxed but ready to pounce. That was more fun and gave me another way of "being" versus just turning up the volume on my own patterns. I felt vulnerable, especially when I first started the neurofeedback. Even though I tried to stay in a good mood, my life wasn't going all that well.

Elsa assured me my brain would figure it out. My job was to be curious about how I felt when the thermometer came down. Breathe and observe.

Over time, I became more successful at adjusting my brain waves to make the thermometer stay down or to be successful at whatever games we were playing. While Elsa, her interns, and I referred to our work as "playing," my brain was the one on the line.

Overall, it was like learning to adjust a lever I didn't even know I had. There were so many frustrating moments in which I tried to create different brain states so I could get a reward. I l-o-v-e rewards. Everyone does, right? For example, when my brain waves were doing what Elsa wanted, the little Pacman would move along nicely, gobbling up the monsters. When my brain was not, Pacman would sit and spin stupidly... over and over.

The training is based on a principle called "operant conditioning." This is exactly what's used to train animals at Sea World or any adult at an ATM. Correct behavior (jumping out of the water at Sea World, entering a password at the ATM) gets the rewards (fish, cash). Moving the Pacman was my reward for producing more adaptive brain waves. My brain was the joystick.

HRV breathing and EEG-based brain training were my main training tools to start. Through repetition, my injured brain became unstuck from the unhealthy patterns it had developed and demonstrated new flexibility. With each major shift in brain waves, my mood and cognitive skills improved. Over time, working through the layers of recovery, I improved my sense of self and my ability to focus, read, drive, and concentrate on the world around me. My physical balance and stamina, memory, and speech fluency also improved. People told me I stopped talking as slowly and was more present, as opposed to being lost in my head.

Cranial Electrotherapy Stimulation (CES)

I was often the first patient of the day and typically got to Elsa's office a little early. By the way, this was totally out of pattern for me to get places early; this commitment felt different. I would sit in the waiting room while the staff set up the clinic. The staff would weave in and out of the waiting room, preparing for the day, arranging magazines, getting the mail and packages. During that time, I noticed they often had something clipped on their ears and carried what looked like a little Walkman for playing CDs. I asked about it, and they said the small machines made them feel great.

As my brain got better, and I could see myself and my life more clearly, I started to experience some level of depression. It was like: "Is this really my life? What am I doing with all this time not working? What am I doing with my life?" The increased cognitive clarity, lack of fogginess, created an emotional depression since I was living more in a broader reality of my life. I had been injured, and the life I knew before had come to a curious standstill I hadn't properly noticed.

After three months, when we did a brain scan (referred to as a "map") update, Elsa said I could benefit from CES. I was excited that I had somehow progressed to using a new tool but didn't know anything about CES. She explained CES stood for cranial electrical stimulation. It didn't hurt. You could barely feel it and was done with that same little device I saw her staff wearing. Elsa explained her CES device, called Alpha-Stim, is used for anxiety, insomnia, and depression. Because I had been struggling with depression, they loaned me one of the units for the weekend.

The instructions were easy: Moisten a little cushion on the ear clip with an electrical-friendly solution and then adjust a small micro-current to a level where I'd feel a little tingle but not feel dizzy or "high."

I tried it at home the next morning while making an early call to my mother in Michigan. I thought, *Why not?* I hadn't told my mother much about my injury or treatment. I know that may sound strange, but I wasn't sure she'd understand or care that much. My life and recovery were all in another world from where she lived. I lived near a big city while she lived in a small town where at that time, you would never have been able even to find a neurotherapist like Elsa. My mother rarely went to doctors because she didn't like to think about herself that much. I could hardly understand what had happened to me, myself, and I couldn't fathom trying to explain my situation to my mom. I was sure I would end up feeling guilty because I felt foggy and overwhelmed much of the time, couldn't keep track of my keys, and couldn't make myself read my Christmas cards until February. This injury was beyond my mom's understanding—as it was mine, at times.

Although my mother was a resourceful and powerful woman who did many kind things for many people, she and I never had an easy relationship—lots of tension and conflict just beneath the surface. But she was my mom. I loved her, and calling regularly was part of my job as a daughter who lived out of town. She also was an early riser and kept herself busy during the day. An early call was perfect. I could check in to see how she was doing before the day got started. However, I didn't have to talk with her too long because we both had things to do. If the CES device made people feel better, it was made for my early morning call with my mom.

It was seven thirty when I clipped the CES onto my ears. I didn't feel anything at first. I kept it on for twenty minutes and didn't sense anything special happening during that time. Sitting in the office in my condo, I found myself staring at some little dust bunnies on the hardwood floor. I hadn't noticed them before. With the phone to my ear, I got up and went to the kitchen for the little dustpan and hand sweeper. I scooped up dust around the office floor while talking to my mom. Then after twenty-five minutes on the phone, I hung up with my mother, having had a fairly pleasant conversation, and went into the bathroom. Even though I had been in and out of the bathroom all day yesterday and the day before, I suddenly noticed the mirror needed a little Windex. I cleaned the mirror.

Then it hit me. Okay, this is weird. It's 7:55 in the morning, and I'm cleaning my house? What? This never happens. And I feel pretty good today. Something's definitely going on here!

I learned this is how brain training works. There is no flashing alert or sign announcing the good changes or how it happened. There are only new instructions from the brain. Using the GPS analogy from Chapter One, the brain won't say: "Hey! Thanks for the great boost of alpha waves. I really needed those to feel better."

Instead, it gives us new messages because we're coming from a different place. New activities and perspectives. When depression and anxiety are lower, we can see outside of ourselves better and focus on the things around us, like the little dust bunnies growing in my home office. One way I noticed changes in my brain was to be aware of the shifts in my perspective, like noticing pictures on the wall in my therapist's office that seemed new but had been there a while. With the CES, I was changing, less concerned on the inside, and able to see the outside more realistically.

I bought my own CES and used it regularly for months. Research continues to show its effectiveness with Post-Traumatic Stress Disorder (PTSD) on returning soldiers, migraines, traumatic brain injury, depression, and anxiety. The cranial electrostimulations device creates a mild stimulation from the battery-operated unit. It is generally imperceptible or gives a slight tingle from the clips on each ear. My acupuncturist, a medical doctor, says this provides a perfect current as it transverses the brain stem. The CES device I used features technology cleared by the FDA to treat anxiety, insomnia, depression, and acute, post-traumatic, and chronic pain.

My personal experience is that this device helped me for a while to feel more alert and positive. However, it wasn't a tool I needed forever. After a certain point using the CES, I really couldn't see any further improvements in my thoughts or behaviors. When we updated my next brain scan, it showed that I had a higher percentage of alpha waves than the normative sample, which can make a person more anxious. That made sense because I had begun to feel my anxiety increase. I would use the CES again in a second if I needed it. I'm glad I have the device. It was a helpful investment, and I use it occasionally with friends.

Last summer, one of my friends, a professional singer, was almost ready to go on tour when he suffered a concussion. He had fallen backward off a ladder and smacked his head on the floor. Poor guy. He was terribly distracted, unable to focus, confused, fatigued, and depressed. He was a brilliant man who suddenly had serious memory issues such as not remembering his phone, keys, and other things that are important to have with you when you're traveling on tour from city to city outside the country. I spoke with the clinical director at Alpha-Stim, a popular CES device, who helped me create a protocol for my friend to use. For two weeks before his trip, he used the Alpha-Stim intensely and then took it with him. By the time he left, he was feeling and functioning much better. When he came back, he said he was fine, and the trip went off without problems.

If you're thinking of purchasing a device like this to use at home, check with a professional first to make sure it's what you need. This device can seem to have a very subtle impact when it's creating big changes. I'd want those changes to be in the right direction to support your goals.

More Brain Tools

We added more tools as my brain increased resilience. Before that, if we did too much or trained too long, I could feel very tired, irritable, or even depressed. These reactions were typically not during the training itself, but that evening or the next day. It's like the day after pushing yourself through a hard physical workout. In Elsa's lab, there were always new things to try because she was always learning, researching, and trying new tools. More than once, my forty-five-minute appointment would span an hour and a half with me happily doing things like breathing hyperbaric oxygen and playing computer games to improve my brainpower. Anyone around Elsa benefited from her curiosity and tools, from patients to interns, students, and friends. This generosity of spirit is one of Elsa's most outstanding qualities.

Wondrous Cracks of Light

There are so many subtle and yet powerful aspects to changing something as fundamental as our brain. As I said earlier, it's easy for us to miss brain improvements, as well as the injury itself. My overriding refrain was that I just wanted to be okay. I never had much of a way to acknowledge or talk about my limitations with most people I knew. I believe few people really understood my path except my husband.

Some moments stand out in Gary's and my memory. We were in the kitchen one day. He had just explained a plumbing situation in our home and what the plumbing company had told him. I looked at him, waiting for the rest of the explanation about the repair. He looked at me, nodded expectantly, and then blinked. A wave of kind patience came over his face. It struck me as familiar. He reset and started to slowly explain the situation:

"Hon, I called the plumber my friend Tom had suggested..." in a tone you'd use with someone who didn't understand.

In that moment, I recognized it as a kindness he had been using all along. I could now see the edges of where things had been and the difference now that I was healing.

I said, "Gary, I got it. I'm with you. I understand what you're saying."

I feel like crying as I write this because it makes me realize how lonely and frightening it must have been for him having a wife who was lost, couldn't track conversations with clarity, and who often wasn't there when you tried to talk with her.

I was coming home. I was inside myself again. I was clearer, tracking our conversation, and connecting with him better. It was a stunning realization. For me, that incident showed I was changing. I was so glad the neurofeedback was working.

To Those Who Lost People Like Me

Such is the path of anyone who loves someone with brain trauma, including wives of professional football players and families of accident victims. It is a difficult and confusing loss. You lose the person you know in certain ways and, hopefully, eventually, you are fortunate, and he or she returns. You hope.

Of course, I wasn't in a coma or dead, and there are *so* many people with injuries much, much worse than my moderate concussion with post-concussion symptoms. But even with my level of injury, there is no guarantee the person you know will ever be the same after a brain injury of any magnitude. It might be easier to see the differences with a more significant injury. Still, many people have experienced injuries like mine and find the repercussions very confusing. They feel disempowered and scared and act that out in confusing ways— aggression, impulsiveness, large emotional highs and lows. Their families can feel helpless, just like my husband did.

On my journey, there were few guideposts and little information about my symptoms and recovery. I saw well-intentioned medical professionals who gave me the best they had to give. My family doctor was the world's greatest for being right with me and explaining what she knew about the experimental treatments I found and would ask her about. In the moment, it made a world of difference, but I know so much more now about what had happened to me. That's one of the reasons why I am writing this. I want parents, spouses, and friends who either have an injury like this, or know someone who does, to know about corridors of trauma and change, to be more sensitive to the subtleties, and not to blame, get overly impatient, or feel hurt and ignored by the injured person's reactions. There is so much more to these injuries and their aftermath than we've understood so far in medical science. We still have much to learn.

Notice the positive. Celebrate it. Reward effort versus result. Keep the faith. Enjoy the moments. Learn all you can about treatments and consider the tools I have found helpful.

My recovery occurred on many levels and wasn't without complexity. For one thing, as I got better, I had a very strong drive to do something important with my life and wondered if I would ever be able to do that. Time now felt limited, and I wanted to use it well. There was a growing sense of purpose, a calling to be a master trainer, a healer. Like Elsa.

Chapter 8:

The Impatient Patient

The Ritual

After the first year of training, I started to wonder if the neurofeedback sessions were really working. I loved seeing and talking with Elsa, and doing the training had been fun. I could see subtle changes, but I wasn't sure the sessions were having a significant impact on my recovery. There was one thing I was certain of, though: I was hungry afterward.

My beeline: It took five minutes to get from Neuroquest, Dr. Baehr's office on Golf Road, to the bagel shop on the corner of Golf and Forest Preserve Drive. I'd order my usual that went unnoted by the tired-looking man behind the counter who was probably just happy the lunch hour rush was over. After about five minutes in the vacant restaurant, a server would bring me a lovely delicacy: a toasted poppy seed bagel with light butter and cream cheese.

The treat began. The cream cheese melted ever so slightly on the warm, toasted, black-seeded, chewy bread and oozed out of the sides as I bit down—over and over until every single bit was gone. Heaven for the famished one. *How could I be so hungry in the middle of the afternoon?*

I learned later that the mental energy required of the neurofeedback training is equivalent to a physical workout. That certainly explained my hunger reaction.

A Snow Day

I am not one to accept something just because an authority figure or anyone else says it's true. I question a lot of things. Despite my moments of breakthrough, I also often thought I should stop the treatments because I couldn't see a difference.

Looking back, I can see that as I got better, I started to realize I had lost time I would never, ever get back. On a good day, I kept the perspective that things were okay. My life was different from what it had been and different from other peoples' lives. It was like a secret life because I didn't talk about much of it to others. No one would understand that I was still being treated over a year later for my concussion. I didn't want to be sick or injured, and the day trading wasn't something many of my friends or family would likely understand I enjoyed. It was like a big Midwest snow day, where you got to stay home and didn't have regular responsibilities but couldn't do much of one's standard routine. On a bad day, it felt like I was trapped and waiting for something, wasting my time. I had so much more I wanted to do with my life, but I had no idea what that was. And I was afraid of what would happen if I tried. I felt pretty lost whenever I let myself think about it.

Walking with Thich Nhat Hanh

In the summer of 2007, my husband and I attended a six-day retreat in the Rocky Mountains with the Vietnamese Zen Buddhist monk and Nobel-Prize-winning peacemaker, Thich Nhat Hanh. He's the author of countless books on mindfulness, meditation, and peace. It was a powerful experience. For this retreat, Elsa gave me the "go" since my brain was in a better place than it was a year earlier when she had vetoed a different days-long retreat. At that time, my brain already had too much theta (slow wave). When I returned, I told Elsa about how great it was to be in Colorado with the thousand other participants, spending a week in instruction with his devotees and being welcomed into the Order of Interbeing. Every detail of these days was a fascination and privilege—what we ate, how we ate (in silence), the hours of meditation, and lectures. I had been on many great spiritual retreats in my lifetime, but this was truly the most inspiring. I will always remember waking up before sunrise to assemble with the hundreds of other dark silhouettes as we quietly walked in meditation with this humble, beautiful, and wise human. Thich Nhat Hanh loved the morning walking meditation, and I walked with him. It was stunning, momentous, and ordinary all at the same time. No pretense, only humility.

Elsa loved learning about interesting teachers and events, but more than just telling her about my vacation, I had another agenda: I was hinting that I had a real life outside the clinic and before I came to her; that I didn't want to be in rehab forever; and, at that point, believed I probably never needed it anyway. Of course, now we know this mindset fits neatly into the anosognosia framework—lack of self-awareness. Still, I went on to tell her about the two books I read during the trip, hoping she would read them, too. Elsa loves new and exciting books.

Her response stunned me.

"Sounds great. And it's good to see you reading. Do you remember how much reading you were doing when you started treatment?"

Me: "Ah... none."

Elsa: "You said it was hard to concentrate that long, and it gave you headaches."

Snap! She was right. I remember saying I didn't enjoy reading books and preferred magazines. Yes, the headaches. Forgot about those. How could I miss the reading part? I had made progress in small ways; I just couldn't see it on my own; I needed people like my husband and Elsa to hold up the mirror for me.

The Lens of Depression

Like many people who have post-concussion syndrome, I suffered from bouts of depression. I watched enough of Oprah to know that journaling and gratitude provided some relief. Thank you, Oprah. Still, somewhere buried quite deep was the sense that nothing would turn out or make a difference in my life: that I was impotent in terms of making anything happen. I didn't feel strong. Any certainty I ever had about being in control, smarter than anyone, or even smart at all, was thoroughly demolished. These were not hard-held assumptions anymore.

There are many reasons that anyone may experience depression after a concussion. These include the injury itself and corresponding physical changes in the brain. The injury disrupts the level of natural chemicals in the brain, and neurotransmitter levels that assist in the brain cells working optimally become unbalanced. The emotional impact is the loss of control and self-esteem. Other factors unrelated to the injury can contribute to someone experiencing depression after a concussion, like previous injuries, genetic disposition in your family, and family stresses from the loss of income, dreams, and vision. Fortunately, I was less conscious of family stresses of lost income since my husband bore the brunt of that without a mention. We did lose the dream of my first book helping many people. But, when I retreated from the training partnership that was the last thing on my mind.

Depression is a multifaceted condition with physical, psychological, biological, and genetic components. With depression, the cognitive filter we use to see the world is that nothing will make a difference. Repeat that three million times, and that's what it's like to be depressed. For a depressed person, the lens through which you see the world shows that nothing is working, will work, or will make a difference.

If you're depressed, chances are you'll have another way of explaining away your progress, especially since positive brain changes don't arrive in a convenient carton we can easily recognize. Instead, the brain tends to subtly make things work better, much like my own progress was subtle and slow. It's like how archeologists dig through ruins; they proceed slowly, digging in tiny increments, layer after layer of sand until historical secrets are revealed.

Even though my default mode was that I didn't need help, it was scary for me to think I was changing, healing, and almost done. I didn't know what my life would be like without the treatment. I couldn't see a path for myself for a long time, but now an angst about it was brewing within me.

Sabotage and Shame

In September 2007, I was training on a new protocol with one of Dr. Baehr's new interns. Her curly dark hair framed her face like Elsa's, only it was much longer. Her name was Tiffany, and she looked like the pride of anyone's family—so smart, capable, and incredibly young. I wanted to discount her as a trainer since she didn't look old enough to drive. However, watching her eyes, you could see she tracked our conversation very well and was confidently giving me her own assessment beyond Elsa's treatment directions. I felt evaluated... by a teenager. Brain evaluated. Like I was a sick person here for treatment.

Tiffany worked with me on a new protocol to help with sleep problems and depression. I had to close my eyes for this protocol, and when a specific type of brain wave decreased (high beta), I'd receive an audio reward. I'd hear this higher-pitched harmonica sound. The sound meant I was doing a good job.

As Tiffany grabbed her clipboard and left the room, I tried to concentrate to distract myself from the tones. I became determined to make them stop rather than happen. It was hard to do, but I was also trying very hard. A crisp black sleep mask covered my eyes to block out the light. Tears of frustration and anger pooled under my mask. It's silly thinking about it now, but yes, I tried to sabotage my training.

I didn't understand myself very well right then. I just felt sort of like being bad after being good during all this rehab session after session. As I thought further, I realized I didn't want the intern running my training to feel like she was doing a good job. *No tone for you, Little Miss Smart New Intern!*

Okay, I realized, especially later, this was a petty moment on my part. I remember crying and confessing this to my beard-stroking therapist: "Here I am, brain-injured, and she is well and happy and has a career she loves, doing this! It's not fair." He didn't say anything. Just sat quietly, eyes soft, and looked at me.

Yes, I was jealous of her life. But I was also ashamed of how angry and petty I felt. Further, I had never seen myself as "brain-disabled" or even used those words, but there was something about the new interns that gave me a different perspective of myself. Old. Slow. Someone who needed treatment. I didn't want to be hurt or need medical care. I wanted to be okay and have a career like hers, helping others. I wanted to be on the other side of the team wearing a white coat and to feel like I knew what I was doing.

This low point ended up being an opening. My jealousy allowed me to see what I wanted so badly. I was very ashamed, but I learned from it. Our feelings can always teach us about what we want and need. The incident ended up fostering a critical change for me.

Chapter 9:

The Power of Dreams

After the Shame Storm

Shortly after my treatment sabotage "shame storm" (thanks Brene Brown for popularizing this great term), I started to talk with Elsa about my vision of becoming a neurofeedback practitioner. It was time. Something was growing inside me that needed to have a voice. My whole dream was to train and work with Dr. Baehr at Neuroquest, but I didn't tell her all of that right away. Small steps, I figured.

Elsa was calm and deliberate. She said if I wanted to work in neurofeedback, I needed to read the most important books in the field, take formal steps and, in time, become board certified. She said there is an international certifying board for biofeedback, which includes neurofeedback. Qualifying practitioners who complete a comprehensive series of training, case studies, and supervision and pass a three-hour exam earn this certification. I loved the idea of a tangible goal, however far away. Dr. Baehr had gone back to school and gotten her Ph.D. in her fifties, which made her a great role model for me.

From another perspective, this shows the recovery happening in my brain. In concussion, the executive functions of strategic planning, decision-making, focus, and being guided by a bigger vision are often compromised. Mine were. Yet, I am and was a person quite motivated by larger goals as with Tae Kwon Do and writing my first book. After the injury, my focus was narrow, on my concerns in the moment. I couldn't execute that well since I couldn't see ahead to plan or didn't even know what I wanted. This desire, goal, and ability to plan embodied my recovery; I started to see a longer view.

Books, Blueprint, BCIA

Elsa suggested books by John Demos and the Thompsons—Michael Thompson, MD, and Lynda Thompson, Ph.D., Canadian researchers and practitioners well-known in the field. They were friends of Elsa's.

To start, I got a copy of Demos's yellow-covered book. My master's degree is in clinical and counseling psychology, and I am a licensed counselor, but my specialty was the psychology of work, with lots of training in organizational behavior and coaching. Although I had a steep learning curve with brain physiology, as I explored in Chapter Six, I had a hidden passion for anything brain-related long before my current goal. My interest in meditation had also attracted me to a Buddhist retreat with psychologist Daniel Goleman. His work on emotional intelligence is important in leadership development. He is a longtime meditator and was an early writer on the brain and meditation.

The certifying body to become a neurofeedback practitioner, Biofeedback Certification International Alliance (BCIA), had a long list of requirements. It included Didactic Neurofeedback Education— thirty-six hours on their Blueprint of Knowledge areas, mentoring hours with an approved mentor, and passing a three-hour objective examination. Another requirement was to have had ten hours of neurofeedback treatment yourself. I felt good to have already completed one of the requirements from their list. It was fun to have a leg up on something having had over sixty neurofeedback sessions already. I could have even satisfied that requirement for a few other people, too.

Now We're Talking—A Workshop!

Through BCIA, I discovered a five-day workshop with John Demos in Ohio. It was hosted by a BCIA-approved training organization called Stress Therapy Solutions. I was psyched. Nothing sounded better to me than driving even the long and monotonously straight I-80 for six hours, Chicago to Cleveland, on a snowy day in March 2008. I was truly excited.

In a chilly Holiday Inn conference room, I sat totally fascinated for five days. I thought I had already known some things about the brain because I knew, say, that the left brain is logical and analytical, and the right brain is spatial.

The workshop covered content way beyond that. It covered basic neurophysiology and neuroanatomy, instrumentation and electronics, psychopharmacological considerations for training, assessment, neurofeedback research, treatment protocols and training, professional conduct, and current trends in the field.

Because I had been unsuccessful in reading Demos's book (my eyes glazed over trying), my brain quickly filled to the brim. It was one thing to be on the receiving end of the sensors, but learning the international placement chart for sensor location, what each location addressed, how the equipment received the brain signals, and everything else was quite another. It was incredible. I started off saying, "Yes, okay. Makes sense." Every topic held my interest. However, if I'd had to explain it to anyone in my own words, it would have been like, "Um... let me get back to you."

The content washed right over me. I'd understood it, well, for a second. But it didn't sink in. I felt like I had no "pockets" or reference points for the information because I had never had a neurofeedback client or thought much about any treatment other than my own. And I certainly wasn't very objective about my own. My mind changed daily about my progress.

Finding My People

Beyond the information, I connected to the workshop because of the room full of geeky, scientific people with all their questions and stories about clients they obviously cared so much about. It made one thing clear: I was home; these were my people. I loved them, and my heart was full. They were quirky and curious in the same way I am. For example, many of them would be happy reading science books on their vacation.

Participants came from all over the country and many kinds of practices—a physician and her physician husband from Kentucky, a neuropsychologist from Maine, a nurse practitioner from Texas.

My initial claim to fame in this new world was knowing Dr. Elsa Baehr, who, along with Dr. Peter Rosenfeld of Northwestern University, pioneered a training protocol to successfully treat resistant depression (the kind that doesn't respond to anything, including medication). I told the instructor that Elsa had recommended his workshop.

"You're training with Elsa? So lucky!"

"Yes, I am doing the neurofeedback training with her. I had a concussion, and now I'm her patient."

"Oh! Okay."

I was the only patient in the room, but no one seemed to notice or care. In addition to Demos, a very articulate and experienced practitioner was Tom Collura. Tom is a pioneer of neurofeedback, an inventor of the most widely used equipment in the field, and a medical engineer. Most people in my (notice, it became "my") field could listen to Tom talk all day and learn an incredible amount about research (he does a lot) and anything brain-related. He's a true genius and a large, brilliant Greek man full of life and stories. Tom's wonderful wife, Terri, owns Stress Therapy Solutions. He was a speaker at the workshop, along with Demos, and the room was thoroughly engaged on a trip through modern neuroscience for all five days.

Calling Forth the Shameless "Inner Fierce"

With this learning phase, as with Tae Kwon Do or more currently my Hip Hop class (yes, I did finally find the right exercise class fit), I might not have absorbed things immediately. But, I am shamelessly relentless about hanging in there, learning and learning to do it right. That's how I am about the things that matter to me—I WILL get it.

My background in career and executive coaching didn't prepare me much for this work. So, I wanted to overtrain in the neurofeedback specialty and learn from the very best people in the field. I never wanted to feel as though I didn't understand what I was doing or that I wasn't prepared for the role I was taking on. I considered it a huge responsibility and honor to help someone's brain.

I did three separate trainings covering Blueprint of Knowledge for the BCIA exam. One was the one with Demos in 2008. Then I spent eight days training in Canada with the Thompsons in 2009. In 2010, I took an online course with a university covering all the content with regular exams interspersed throughout. These learning opportunities were a dream and I devoured them. It gave my life a strong sense of purpose to learn my new field with the highest competence. Judy Crawford, the executive director of BCIA, said that in preparing for the certification application, I was one of the most conscientious people she had ever seen.

Okay, maybe I was a little obsessive.

In writing this and thinking about my training, I've come to wonder whether we don't all have this "inner fierce" conscientious person inside of us and how important it is. Certainly, I know we all have voices in our heads like the depressed voice ("nothing will make a difference") and the shamed one ("I am bad and stupid; I make mistakes"). But as a coach, I see my work as locating and calling out my clients' "inner fierce" person. I coax and challenge them as I would you: Be diligent and intense; this is your life; determine what you want and work toward it. Even if you don't know your own goals, move in the direction that feels right inside.

Anchoring My Commitment

In the sea of information I was learning and the avalanche of my own new thoughts related to it, three things stood out. They anchored me and made me even more committed to my goal of working with the brain. I felt the stones under my feet. This was my path and the direction I wanted to go with my life.

First, Clarity Breeds Clarity

The workshop gave me insight into hundreds of people I had seen in my career coaching practice. If people are unclear about their career choice, they are often unclear about more than that—their relationships, where they live, etc. I knew that career indecision is complicated, and even after reading excellent books like *What Color is Your Parachute*, some were still stuck. They didn't know their strengths, couldn't decide what would create satisfying emotional employment for them, and couldn't commit to a course of action. That's why I wrote *Back in Control*—to help people master the psychological underpinnings of change. This is important.

Now I see that working with the brain to reduce stress, strengthen confidence after loss or injury, and get clearer in life can all help one's career as well as life. Many stuck people would benefit tremendously from improving how they process information, focus, utilize memory, and exhibit emotional intelligence. These skills would foster being able to create a career/life vision and weather the process of finding the next right work situation.

In fact, my brain training offered these benefits of increased personal clarity of my wants and needs. That provided the most solid evidence that my training was, in fact, working well. I felt clearer.

Many executives I had worked with were stressed, overwhelmed and/or lacked a bigger view of their organization. Many left bodies along the path of their progress and could easily benefit from neurofeedback tools to control their immediate emotional responses.

These tools would make life easier and better for a lot of people. In Chapter Seventeen, I'll share stories with you on the impact of using neurofeedback and other brain-based tools on careers, job performance, parenting and life, overall.

All Brains Crave the Same Thing

A second major takeaway from this first workshop was that whether it's drugs, alcohol, or any other addiction, all anyone wants is to make his or her brain feel normal and good. At the base of it all, that's not a moral or a good versus evil issue. It's someone taking a more or less effective route to mental balance. For example, we reviewed research on the brain scans of alcoholics. They generally showed significant deficits of alpha waves in specific locations. At the right levels, alpha waves help us feel relaxed and a sense of peaceful satisfaction. Alpha waves increase from alcohol intake, so it addresses a need to feel mellow and calm. However, within hours after drinking, another change occurs in the brain. High beta (a faster brain wave frequency) increases to a dysfunctional level, which results in anxiety and irritability. So, in this restless, edgy state, a drink can sound like a good idea, and the cycle begins. While there are other powerful factors like environment and genetics in determining who will become an alcoholic, this biological loop is quite powerful.

All Pain is Brain Pain

Third, the centers of the brain stimulated from physical pain are the same for emotional pain, like depression. In other words, depressed people aren't just trying to annoy others or refusing to see the glass "half full." They are hurting—literally. Baehr and Rosenthal's discovery was that depression coincided with unevenness or asymmetry in the presence of alpha waves across the front of the brain. The left side has too much alpha, which is thought to impact the brain's endogenous reward system that releases neurotransmitters of happiness (dopamine) when we do things like check things off a list, pet small animals, and look at cute babies. On the other side, activities like exercise and psychotherapy help change and normalize the brain and relieve depression.

After I finished my initial thirty-six-credit Blueprint training with John Demos, I debriefed with Elsa, who helped me apply some things I was learning in a way that changed everything.

Chapter 10:

Second Chances

Critical Questions about Life

Reflecting on what happened next makes me ask these critical questions: how many of us give others a second chance at the big things in life? Would you provide another person the opportunity to recover and restart their life anew after a setback, whether you caused it or not? Or does your thinking get stuck in biases and stereotypes? Should the person who naively thought selling pot before it was a viable business option and was busted as a dealer be forever branded as a felon? Is it right that someone who leaves prison, having paid his or her dues, should forever be without meaningful work? Decades after something bad happens, should we let others continue to pay the price without a chance to learn and to do things differently? Do you and I help people create new beginnings from bad judgment, mistakes, or simple accidents? Do we help people overcome the wreckage of the past?

Elsa's Hands

The next steps were in Elsa's hands, and what she did shaped my opportunities. She reached out to friends in her network and asked them if I could volunteer in their neurofeedback practices. I could have never done that on my own. I'd never have figured out who to call. I'd have had a hard time saying, "I'm Diane Wilson. I've been in treatment for neurofeedback with Dr. Elsa Baehr. I'm not a student or graduate student but a middle-lifer recovering from post-concussive syndrome, and would like to sit, watch what you do, learn and help out if I can." That would not have happened or certainly not easily. And even if I did make that phone call, I'm not sure it would have brought me the same opportunities I was given through her outreach. I was lucky. I was lucky to be given a second chance at a full life post-injury and to have the opportunity to learn to become a healer like Elsa.

The Midlife Intern

Beginning in 2008 and for the next two years, I interned. First, I was in the private practice of a busy psychologist treating adults and children, then in a QEEG (Quantitative Encephalogram) assessment department of a hospital for alcohol rehabilitation, and finally, very briefly in a clinic helping autistic children. The managers were all members of a professional organization Elsa belonged to called EEG Chicago based on the work they shared using EEG-based training (neurofeedback). I got to see different practices, meet people who did the work I wanted to do, and see how they treated patients. They were amazing experiences.

I spent the most time in the private practice of Dr. Kathy Abbott, where I went for a day each week for about a year. Dr. Abbott, a psychologist, is a devoted teacher of neurofeedback and had a big practice in the south suburbs of Chicago and in Oak Park. At that point in her career, she saw patients six days a week. She is a walking encyclopedia of studies in the field on a range of conditions she treats—ADHD, autism, addiction, learning disabilities, work stress, depression, and mild traumatic brain injury. Her Oak Park office was in the Rush Hospital professional suites because she had been on staff in their alcoholism unit before going into private practice. My role was to clean the sensors, paste them to the proper spot on a patient's head, and generally help in any way I could. Dr. Abbott was always there and loved chatting with everyone.

It struck me how genuine her interest was by how she treated patients when she saw them in the waiting room. I wondered if week after week the pleasantries would become boring.

"Hello, Joey! How ARE *you* today? Hello, Sara! How's Joey's *mom* today?"

I hope to always like my clients that well and convey to them how invested I am in our work. Like Drs. Baehr and Abbott, I think good therapists in this field are pretty geeky (everything comes back to the brain), and they truly enjoy their work. As a patient going once or twice a week, I experienced my own high and low periods. A therapist's enthusiasm is like the grease on the skids to move you forward.

Dr. Abbott is well-connected in the learning circles of neurofeedback and always knew what key people in the field were doing or finding in their research. She often fine-tuned her training protocols and bought new equipment with different capabilities based on what she was learning. You can feel how close-knit the field of neurofeedback is when talking with her because she's developed relationships with thought leaders in the field and consults with them regularly on patient issues. She's always learning. She's been active in a key neurofeedback organization called the International Society for Neurofeedback Research (INSR) and has served on their Board of Directors.

At first, the nuances of the brain training were lost on me. Because even after the five-day training in Ohio, I hardly had any idea of what Dr. Abbott was talking about most of the time. I didn't even know which questions to ask. She was passionate about her patients, and I was happy to absorb whatever I could. But I dreamed of the day I would have a better understanding of the world of EEG-based brain training. It was like sitting through a lunch with nice people you didn't know who spoke a different language. You just absorb what you can, trusting you'll learn as you go along. Dr. Abbott has great instincts about which brain waves each client needs more of, less of, how to balance them, and the training strategies to make this happen.

Here's an example of an early conversation with Dr. Abbott about a little boy's training. He's sweet, but the class clown and impossible to settle down and do his schoolwork. Mom is extremely concerned about him getting through the third grade.

"We're using this 60% reinforcement schedule to reduce theta at FZ so that he'll be able to pay attention better at school. We'll decrease theta in the front and later increase theta and alpha in the back at OZ. This will help his sleep be deeper and more restorative."

"Great, I'll go get him from the waiting room." I would have no idea what we were doing, but I was happy to greet him and his mom.

I loved the families we saw and truly enjoyed my time with Dr. Abbott (who shortly preferred I call her Kathy). We've remained colleagues and friends long after my internship ended in 2009. In recent years, we've had a couple of brain geek days holing up in her office to discuss what's working with our clients, what we're learning from our reading, new training equipment, and our husbands. We try new protocols on and do QEEGs on each other. Only someone as passionate about neuroscience as I am could possibly grasp how happy those days make me feel and how grateful I am to have her in my life. I will always be grateful for her mentorship especially in the early days of my new career.

Bonus Feedback

Kathy was always a good observer and held a unique role in commenting now and then in ways that helped me understand how I was doing.

"You seem much more tuned in now than when you first started with me," she told me one day when I was her intern. "Your attention span is longer, and you're able to make decisions faster. You noticed that Sam was able to stay with the game longer, and I didn't catch that. You were right. Two sets of eyes are better than one, and that was a good insight you had about why Sam won't wear his helmet at school when he should be." *Great!*

You get the idea. Our time together had a nice blending of professional and personal feedback at points in a world that doesn't give much brain function feedback.

Brain function is such an odd area of life. As adults, we don't get much (or any) personal feedback from others on how our brain is working. That leaves many of us hoping we haven't made a mistake or come up short. I've noticed as people get older (myself included), we can feel self-conscious about our age and thinking we are slow when, in fact, we are not. It's a quirky area. Before my concussion, when I felt good about how my brain worked, no one ever said: "Man! She is so smart," or anything like that—except in grade school when my teachers always gave good feedback. During this stretch of brain challenge, very few people ever said to me: "Hard day, huh?"

However, if my hairstylist somehow clipped a little too much off during the regular eight-week trim, I'd get tons of comments like:

"New hair cut?"

"Hair looks different."

That's difficult since I have spent hours and hours and hours trying to heal and optimize my brain. It's the same for my clients.

I'll say: "Do you get any feedback at work about how you're doing? You said you're less likely to jump in during department meetings before you've thought your comments through and are more able to listen to others."

"Nope."

This lack of feedback is why in executive coaching coaches often design projects to collect feedback from their client's boss, peers, and co-workers.

My regular clinic day with Kathy usually ended with date night with my husband at our favorite Thai restaurant, The King and I, in Oak Park. It was so special to meet after my day "at work." I would be nicely dressed and feel fully justified in ordering a meal. Sitting across the table, I would tell my husband about what we did that day and this amazing work. Never names. Confidentiality is always observed.

For example, I might explain how Client X raised his D to a B on his report card. And how the stressed executive decided to give up her sleep medication since she didn't need it anymore. Or how we did 4-channel, Live Z-score training on Dr. Abbott's new Brain Avatar.

I would pour over the menu but almost always order the same thing—Crab Rangoon, veggie fried rice, and extra sweet and sour sauce. The creamy cheese oozed out when I took a bite of the crusty Crab Rangoon. We savored each one, and the standard appetizer Rangoon count was six. It was a quiet time in the restaurant business cycle, and the servers came to know us. I felt proud for having a full workday in my new field even though I was a volunteer and mainly watched the treatments and cleaned the sensors between patients. It was still good work.

There were many good days during this period of 2008, but I also struggled with depression and a deep sense of helplessness. Life had shifted so quickly; my footing was shaky. I struggled with feeling lost, disconnected, and in the end, as if nothing would make a difference.

Then the stock market crashed. It left the outside world of finance and anything related to banking and money in a state of chaos that matched my deepest insides.

Join a ... What?!

One day, when life seemed at an impasse on so many levels, we decided to join the church at the end of our block, Unity Temple. We had always loved it from the outside. I love beautiful architecture, and the building is a historical landmark designed by Frank Lloyd Wright. I had been talking with our neighbor, Tom, whose wife was gone on a writing retreat with a Unity Temple group she had been writing with for many years. It sounded like such a comfort and sort of like a coconut falling from the sky. I talked to my husband, and we decided to try the church out.

My husband and I are not joiners, much less church joiners. Before that talk with Tom, we worshipped Sunday morning coffee, thick newspapers, and news programs sitting in our pajamas until noon. Heaven. We also occasionally meditated at a Thai Buddhist temple and just loved that Thai community.

But it felt like big things in the life I had known had changed; I thought maybe it would be nice to belong to a church like so many other people did. Not to mention, it offered a chance to fulfill a dream I had always had. All my life, I had wanted to learn to sing and to have time for it. If life could change in an instant, why not learn to sing?

Don't worry. I promise this won't get too churchy. But from the first service, I felt like being a Unitarian was a good idea. It embodied many things I believed and didn't pretend to have all the answers, except to build community. Here is the convenant repeat each service:

"Love is the doctrine of this congregation,
The quest of truth is its sacrament,
And service is its pray
To dwell together in peace,
To seek knowledge in freedom,
To serve human need,
To the end that all souls shall grow into harmony with the Divine —
Thus do we covenant with each other and with God."

— Arranged by L. Griswold Williams

Unity Temple is inclusive. You could be a Catholic, a former Catholic (like me), Jewish, agnostic, or from anywhere else and still be a member. They have many social action programs, like helping the homeless in our area and fighting for those whose rights are being threatened. It is a working community of people, and there were so many activities going on that I could volunteer until my schedule was full. Unitarians don't argue dogma. They accept others, even those very unlike them. They roll up their sleeves to work at making the world a fairer and more just place. It wasn't about allegiance to any specific doctrine of faith other than acceptance and love for others.

The Mystery and Belonging

The one activity I got involved in right away was the choir. One evening, Tom introduced me to the charismatic and elegant choir director before rehearsal started, and she was welcoming. She asked me to sing for her while she played notes on a lovely grand piano in the sanctuary. My only singing had been in the shower or after three hours on a car ride to Michigan when I was totally out of things to talk about with my husband. The Jewel and Joni Mitchell moments.

After I sang, she had me sit in a specific section of the choir. From the beginning, I loved singing. I had no idea how to produce the right sound by looking at the notes on the page, but I somehow did. It's a God thing. I had never been in a choir before that. I played clarinet and mostly twirled baton in high school and took dance classes in college. It was like an envelope of safety in the company of nice people. My injury and treatment had been so isolating. My coaching practice was very part-time with only two or three clients, and when I did work with clients, I worked alone.

Finally, I had a place to belong.

As I look back, ten years later, having learned what I learned over the years and continue to learn about key signatures, rhythms, and sounds, I have no idea how I participated and loved it so much when I knew so little. The music we sing is sophisticated. I guess I thought it would be hymns and popular tunes. Sometimes it is, but we also sing in French, Latin, and Yiddish. We sing Mozart masses and other complex pieces. Our twice-yearly singing major events are accompanied by an orchestra. Many members of the choir have sung their whole lives, and for some of them, that's a long time.

I loved music, but I never considered myself a musician. Having no idea what I sounded like, I started as a second alto, the lowest of the female voices. During the first season, I moved up to the first alto group because my voice was higher than the seconds. Still, during rehearsal, I would listen to the light, high, heavenly voices of the soprano section and long to sing like that. I couldn't imagine how life would feel if I could make sounds like that.

Before one of the major works the choir performed at a big event, we had a chance to share in the service during a segment called Joys and Sorrows. The date coincided with the period that my neurofeedback treatment was (finally) ending with Elsa.

I felt shy, but I stepped up to the microphone in the sanctuary. I expressed how grateful I was to the choir and choir director because singing in the choir was one of the few areas of my life where I felt like I could do something that turned out well. I told the congregation that I had had a concussion and brain injury but was happy to be near the end of my treatment. Unity had been a safe place for me; singing had helped me heal my brain. I was nervous, but my speech turned out beautifully, and people were crying. No one in the choir had known about my injury before that. I didn't know many people personally because our time together was focused on singing, and I didn't like to talk about it. This was a major step for me to be honest about who I was and where I had been. I felt safe.

Music Heals

I never wanted our Wednesday night choir rehearsals to end. I would look at my watch and hate that the time had gone so fast. In bed afterward, I felt like every single cell of my being was happy in a way it hadn't been in a long time, or maybe ever. The music we sang played over and over in my head the rest of the night. It was so wonderful to be one of a group that included such talented people from different worlds and lives coming together to make something so special.

I believe music helped heal my brain. I know that in my soul. Music makes everything better. I read that music allows groups of people singing together to develop a synchrony of brain wave patterns. If so, for me, this synchrony seemed to stretch and uncoil some of the stuck patterns of my injured brain. I became more positive, energized, and flexible with life.

Music perception, governed by the right brain, is mystical. I have no idea how I can find a pitch so easily. I just know what it sounds like in my head. A choir mate once told me when we start out singing new music, she often gets the pitch from hearing me. I don't know what specific notes named "A-flat" or "C-sharp" would sound like, but my body knows. To sing, I have to lend myself to the mystical because it defies rational thought and activity. I believe music and love are intertwined when I sing with the choir. It is through music that my brain became whole and created space for other things to grow. With time and lessons, I also discovered my natural vocal type. It turns out my vocal range is wide, being able to sing low as well as very high notes. For me, that means, I actually get to sing with those heavenly first sopranos. Pretty cool, huh?

Looking back, it's as though music and the choir created big stones just beneath the surface of the deep water. Grounding pieces to my life. We had followed what seemed like random activity—joining a church that had been at the end of the block even before I moved there (ten years earlier). These stones became a healing path as I trusted myself to follow my intuition and explore. As remarkable as walking across a lake, the random steps created new neural pathways within a brain that was slowly and steadily finding its way to becoming whole again.

The Testimonial

A few weeks after the big music event, I was invited to give a brief testimonial in front of our congregation about my membership and what it meant to me. In my professional life, I was a skilled public speaker. On my book tour, I had done over thirty-five radio and television interviews about issues related to work transition. I was lucky enough to be on major stations like CNN, ABC, NBC, and public radio in Chicago, Wisconsin, and Michigan. So, part of me understood the role of public speaking. However, it was easier to talk about a book I wrote to help others than to speak about my life, my brain, and what my church had meant to me.

I had ten minutes.

In gratitude, I said I could have healed on my own, but instead of being alone and healed, I was given the opportunity and support to learn to sing and be healed. I went on to explain that that there was something bigger in this story than my own brain.

Grandma Grimard

Growing up, my father's mother, Grandma Grimard, lived far away from us. Originally from England, she had emigrated from Canada with her French-Canadian husband, and after having the last of her ten children, she had a stroke. It paralyzed her left side, and she could no longer talk. She could only say one word, and she repeated it over and over.

Throughout her life, she continued to play the violin, even after the stroke. When she visited from Colorado and stayed with us, she would need to practice. Even at ninety-four years old, she still took violin lessons. As kids, we would peek curiously into the doorway and then run away. As a little girl, I could see that even though she could no longer sing, her body could. With a music stand in front of her, she would wedge the violin under her chin over her stiff left side, stroke the bow with her right arm, and hum from deep within. She felt the music that played inside her. This beautiful image of my strong and spirited Grandma Grimard is emblazoned into my being.

It's a small detail and might be hard to understand logically. When the choir participates in services where we are listed in the program individually, we are always asked if our name is listed and spelled correctly. My family (Grimard) accompanies my married last name and is the longest among the female singers. I pause because I'm aware of that and don't want to stand out. Still, I always list my name as Diane Grimard Wilson. To me, it's a way of including my grandma. I am the lucky one who got to sing. I am singing for her. Always.

So, I shared all of that. The church testimony I gave was powerful for others and for me. I hadn't talked much about my life and injury. After I walked home from Unity Temple that day, I sat on the couch. And that's where I stayed. I stared straight ahead for the rest of the afternoon—mind blank, no thoughts, body frozen. I didn't move. I couldn't.

Chapter 11:

Just When I Thought
I Was Done!

Understanding Injury

When I talked with Dr. Locke, I told her about what happened after my testimony at Unity Temple. I wasn't concerned about much of my behavior since the accident. I didn't worry about myself that much. But it was even strange to me that after my talk, I just sat in the living room, staring, the rest of the afternoon.

"Your brain injury is no longer the issue," she said. "Your brain is pretty much healed."

This made no sense to me until she added this last word:

"Physically."

"What you are experiencing isn't the brain injury. Instead, the issue is brain trauma."

Trauma was never a word I had associated with my car accident. By definition, trauma means "a deeply distressing or disturbing experience." (Google)

Yet, it did fit.

It felt innovative to have had neurofeedback treatment for the concussion and post-concussion symptoms. But it was intriguing and disappointing to think that this was the emotional reaction of a traumatized person –defining, and yet another challenge I would have to work through. It did, however, help me make sense out of a lot of things I hadn't put together—emotional numbness, preoccupation, and intense emotional responses. These symptoms didn't sound like me, but they were occurring. I couldn't deny it. It was like the plumber who has leaky pipes in his or her own home. And, it was disappointing because I just wanted to be okay.

The testimonial at church had been a turning point. It triggered me, but it also helped me see the intensity of my reaction—my numbness and staring the rest of that afternoon.

It was helpful to have my kind husband there, who was so supportive as I realized how traumatized I was. Many people aren't that lucky. Their actions have already alienated the people closest to them. We reflect on that time now, and he says he felt pretty helpless. I think families of people going through injury and trauma are often the biggest heroes. My husband didn't sign on for any of this; he was helpless. He had a wife who'd incurred a condition that at least initially changed everything, with no name for it and very outside support in dealing with it. He probably wondered a lot about what life would be like for us from there on. Then, after describing my healing to my church with such gratitude, I sat still and numb the rest of the day.

Events like talking about the accident triggered the emotional responses I had at the time. My brain was unable to process the deeply disturbing emotions in that situation. They were stuck in my brain, and I replayed them in situations that were triggers. When I was triggered, my brain experienced the awfulness of the injury on an emotional level.

Licensed in the field of mental health, I did some research and talked to a close friend who is also a therapist. We determined that the best route going forward was to seek treatment for the emotional trauma itself.

At the same time, a new career coaching client of mine mentioned he had been in New York City near the Twin Towers on 9/11 and that he and many people he knew had gone through a series of

EMDR sessions to help eradicate the devastating grip of seeing and experiencing the loss and destruction. It's often the case that the answers to questions I'm thinking about for myself or a client comes from someone completely unrelated or unknowing of the issue.

EMDR had piqued my curiosity.

The acronym stands for *eye movement desensitization and reprocessing*. It's a powerful technique based on the premise that with trauma, like an accident or bombing, the brain is unable to process the memory. It is too traumatic, too overwhelming to digest. These memories then get stuck, and when things trigger a recall of the event, the brain will respond as though it was experiencing the very same situation, with all the same protective responses—fight, flight and/or freeze. A soldier home from a war zone with PTSD might hear a car on the street backfire and respond exactly like he would have on the battlefield: intense fear, running, or readiness to fight. The nervous system gets stuck in high gear with these potentialities in the moment. Everyday events triggering this kind of fear exact a toll on our resources (stress) and keep us from living in the present for conversations, work, and creativity.

Psychologist Francine Shapiro, who originated EMDR, found that these memories can be "processed" later by helping the brain do so. By accident, she discovered that the back and forth rhythmic movement of her fingers in front of a patient's eyes somehow created a path for the memories to replay and be consolidated in the memory system of the person. The emotions lose their intensity, and perspective is created in terms of time and social context.

You can finally say to yourself: "This happened. It was awful, but it's over. I survived. I am a survivor. I am not alone. I have people who loved and love me."

Through this, we are no longer plagued by instinctual reactions to events from another time. Sounds amazing, right? Thank you, Francine Shapiro.

This made sense of the numbness I had after talking at my church. So, I decided to do some sessions with a trained EMDR therapist.

As therapy tools go, EMDR is a highly controlled technique. In my research, it became clear some people really knew EMDR and were well-trained, and as a person with a rather significant vulnerability, that's what I wanted. I would want the very same for you.

Thanks to Lord Google, I found EMDRia. It is an organization Shapiro started that offers EMDR training to therapists and a listing of providers trained and certified by the organization. As a therapist, I know this is not something you can learn in a weekend workshop or by reading a book. Similarly, as a patient, this can be a very discrete sequence of sessions that you go through to address your concern. It doesn't have to be open-ended and unending. The client from New York City I mentioned had just twelve sessions.

That gave me a sense of mission.

I Need a Driver Again!?

The EMDR therapist I saw was certified by EMDRia and about an hour from my home. When scheduling my appointment, she told me I would need to have someone drive me home afterward. Of course, that scared the daylights out of me. Not to mention that I had already lost four months of driving due to the accident.

I saw her about six times. It turned out there were other concerns in the picture that I hadn't recognized until I did this treatment.

Again, funny how we stop seeing—and even normalize—the most abnormal things. For example, when riding in the car as a passenger, I would often start screaming and yell "STOP!" because I thought cars were going to hit us. I couldn't help myself. I'm serious. To me, it was real. But my husband is a great driver (usually), and I was super-sensitive. It wasn't until after my church testimonial that I saw myself as having PTSD, and I started to link little curious aspects of my behavior to it.

The other thing was whenever I talked about the accident, I felt emotional, like I was going to cry. No wonder I didn't talk about it with people. Who would want to be taken out of normal life to talk about something that almost always makes you choke up when you are doing it?

You may read these examples and wonder if I thought either was "normal" behavior. When you go through something like this, you don't think about the things you do as being normal or not. You're just trying to get through the day. It was what it was. I was the way I was. You stop measuring yourself against "normal." This was my life.

A notable example: For the legal aspects of the accident, I had to sit for a deposition with my lawyer, a court reporter, the driver's lawyer, and for some reason, the person who drove into me. Poor guy, he looked so uncomfortable. My job was to answer questions about what had happened. During the first part of the questioning, I didn't cry. My face did, though. Tears streamed down my face almost the whole interview. It was embarrassing and horrible. I couldn't stop it. Not for my life. It was just short of four years after the accident itself, and I sincerely tried to keep it together. It was one of the most difficult things I ever went through in my whole life. I just couldn't stop crying.

EMDR Sessions

My EMDR therapist was careful, kind, and methodical. In the intake session, she asked questions about what happened, how I felt, my life, and my personal history. Over the following few sessions, she took me through a series of activities to see how best to do the procedure and then addressed the key issues.

There are different ways to activate the processing of the stuck emotional data besides eye movements and finger-waving (which made me dizzy). She also had a stand about five feet high, which looked like a small windmill with a three-foot bar across the top, covered with small twinkly lights that spun around in front of me. That wasn't going to work for me either. I felt queasy at the thought of watching the bar of lights spin in front of me. In the end, we used these little walnut-sized shells or orbs that I tucked into each hand. They vibrated at different speeds the therapist controlled.

It was easiest for me to close my eyes (an option), and the therapist would ask me questions about what happened, how I felt, my most troubling sensory reactions, and triggers of the intense responses I was having. Holding these little orbs, I would visualize the scenes. The shells would vibrate, and I would sit still and feel the vibration until the scene disappeared or something changed in it. She would intervene and ask what was happening for me. At first, I felt hopeless at the process and thought it wasn't going to help at all. I would visualize the accident and the scene, but then my mind would drift off. But I fessed up and told the therapist that my mind was drifting. She said something like: "What did you see when you drifted off?"

"Oh, I started thinking about my dad and how much I love my dad."

"Okay."

It was the kind of approving "okay" that makes you think maybe you're not screwing it up. Her "okay" made me believe that somehow, I was doing a decent job at being a trauma patient on the road to recovery.

After drifting off the next time, I learned to be curious about where my mind and body reactions went. Everything meant something. For example, finding the psychic protection of my dad in my brain as I processed the accident was important—the bigger context was that I was loved. Feeling that is an emotional resource. With my own clients, sometimes we need to build emotional resources they can feel before we work on processing trauma. We all come from our own paths.

The EMDR process was sometimes like having an emotional fever that built up and then broke. Still, it never felt overwhelming to me. I was curious and amazed to see and feel what drifted in and out of my mind and body. But it was also hard. I recalled and re-experienced difficult aspects of being injured that I had forgotten but were still sitting in my brain, draining my energy. Eventually, I could feel the changes from EMDR inside. I felt more present as if the emotional wounds in my life hidden under the bandages were healing.

The Legal Issue

At one point early in the EMDR treatment, my husband and I needed to make a decision. The suit with the driver's insurance company was potentially going to court. And EMDR is likely to change the emotions a person has about an accident, which affects how they will appear in court. With good treatment, you will appear less emotionally vulnerable and damaged by what happened. Some people may want to simply testify about what the accident did to them, not how they are after being treated with a powerful tool like EMDR.

In EMDR, if a therapist is treating someone in this situation, it is important for there to be a conscious decision about the treatment. When it looked like I would have a court hearing, we (my husband and I) still chose to do this treatment. I wanted the grip of this accident off me, whether I made a compelling witness for a settlement or not.

The outcome of my EMDR sessions was positive. While initially, I didn't understand why I needed someone to drive me home, I quickly saw why. After most sessions, I felt thick, dreamy, dazed, and preoccupied. My reaction time for managing a car going sixty miles an hour down an expressway was not where it needed to be. My therapist said that free association writing (writing whatever came to mind) would help accelerate the process. She said that if I felt scared or overwhelmed by anything that popped up in my mind in the days afterward, I could call her. That was comforting—and scary—at the same time. Luckily, no pieces of loosened traumatic memory emerged between sessions.

Did EMDR work? Yes.

EMDR is an amazing therapy. I think I could have used a few more sessions, but the woman I was working with took a job in a hospital and was no longer available. On the positive side, it gave me more of an internal sense of feeling solid. I no longer spontaneously yell in the car in needless fear. I almost forgot I used to do that. I feel calmer and clearer in a way that is deep and hard to describe. Clearing this emotional underbrush away helped me be more present. I can see other people and outside situations much more clearly. My deep internal fear had kept me self-focused and overly self-protective? I gained more capacity and energy for life outside of myself.

Training the Therapist

After my personal EMDR experience, my friend Mary (also a therapist) and I decided to get trained in EMDR. Because having personal experience with EMDR was one of the certification requirements, I felt like I had a leg up again. It was nice to be ahead on something. Training as therapists and coaches almost always entails using the techniques on ourselves first. My own trauma treatment qualified me.

Mary was so eager to find a workshop offered by EMDRia that she traveled to another city for one and told me later what happened. That only convinced me further that EMDR was an amazing tool.

Buried Trauma

An incredible person and gifted therapist, Mary would describe herself as a weird kid—sort of bookish, socks didn't always match, and socially awkward. Growing up in Arizona, her mom suffered from a significant mental illness and then died when Mary was ten. So, she had to learn many things about life on her own, plus deal with a very unstable home with two wild brothers and an explosive father. School was hell; the other kids made fun of Mary but even more traumatic, so did her teachers. These are the kind of life experiences that can either make someone into an extremely sensitive person, one who can imagine any difficult situation her clients have been through, or a huge bully herself. Mary has that sensitivity and ...is an exceptional therapist. Still, these humiliating memories lived buried in her psyche.

At that time, therapists learned and practiced EMDR techniques on each other for three days straight. Intense.

In training, therapists use real material and put themselves into the process. There are guidelines on who can participate in the training. If you have experienced recent trauma or are in therapy (like most good therapists are), you needed to have your therapist's approval to commit to this. Mary did the first two days of training with no major personal reaction or insights.

She sent me a note: "No biggie here, not sure what this does."

After the second training day, in her hotel room, Mary took a shower. Under the steady water sprinkling on her head, something strange happened. It was like someone had taken a brick out of the wall of memories, revealing the wall of hurt and deep anger she had buried.

She heard this: "They didn't know what they were doing. They just didn't know."

From that evening forward, Mary had a shift of perspective. She no longer viewed those childhood scenes only from the angle of a kid. She could see them from a higher level, with a wider lens. She no longer felt like the victim of ridicule and bullying in school. She felt sorry for any teacher who would pick on a small child and came to believe the kids in her class were as lost as she was in some ways. She had a huge wave of compassion for everyone in the situation, as well as for herself as a beautiful, awkward little girl with no mom.

In the months that followed, Mary surprised herself by going to one of her high school class reunions for the first time. There she talked to people who were surprised to see her. Some of them even confessed face to face how sorry they were for how they treated her. She had forgiven them long ago but at the reunion was able to tell them she did. She was no longer a lost child or a victim. Anyone could see that. Her barriers were down, and she reached out.

Mary formed new relationships with these old classmates who had gone through the pains of grade school with her in this small town. They still keep in touch.

I always tell my EMDR clients Mary's story. Changes from EMDR can come in many ways. Mine were more incremental—small pieces with some fevers and a burst. But Mary's was a major gestalt shift.

I have completed the basic level of EMDR training, which took a year of sequenced workshops with hours of supervision and case review. I still have much to learn about it and hope to train to work with more complex cases. For now, I am comfortable with my skill level for the people I see but don't hesitate to seek supervision from a more seasoned EMDR therapist if I need it.

I generally love the EMDR work I have done to help clients. I have witnessed them move past traumas like loss, accidents, and assaults to one's sense of self, such as physical and psychological abuse. EMDR is also useful with non-trauma goals like helping peak performers move beyond past beliefs that interfere with their success in sports or work. It wouldn't be the only new tool I needed to help me.

Chapter 12:

About That Bagel

Food Power

Before finishing my treatment with Elsa in June 2009, she helped me with a significant discovery. Her insights on the influence of food on the brain were constantly growing. In the throes of also caring for her ailing and beloved husband, Rufus, she was a learning machine about everything that affected the brain and body.

I, too, had started to wonder about the impact of the food I was eating on my healing and health. It proved quite difficult to track my emotions and how my brain was getting me through my reactions and life overall. Was there a food that was contributing to my feelings of being foggy, scattered, and unmotivated? If so, what was it?

With Elsa's support, I made an appointment to have food sensitivity testing done with a doctor. The results were stunning. The three pages listed sixty-four foods with a red bar next to each, which indicated a food sensitivity. The length of the red bar across the page was the index of the degree of food intolerance. My results pages had long red horizontal lines across it. Lots of long red lines. In other words, I was highly sensitive to tons of foods. You know that toasty poppy seed bagel (wheat)? The melted butter (dairy)? Cream cheese (dairy)? Crispy Crab Rangoon (wheat and dairy)? All, not so good for my brain and body. *Oh my gosh!*

Test Results

My sensitivities included every major category of food you probably love, and certainly that I did. The big ones were dairy (particularly the milk protein, casein), wheat, soy, peanuts, corn, orange juice (OJ?), and eggs. There were others, too, like garlic, cherries, and asparagus. As I look back, I now realize how my relationship with these foods manifested itself in my attention and focus, but I had no idea at the time. It wasn't as easy as tracking one food and its effects because there were so many irritants for me. Some had a delayed effect, days later, and others were immediate.

They were all innocently and even ceremoniously wrapped into my life. For example, now and then, my husband and I used to love to go out for Sunday brunch. I'd order my favorite breakfast: an omelet, potatoes, juice, and toast with lots of butter. It was delicious. Then I'd typically go home, hit the couch for a bit, put pillows under my knees to elevate them, and read the Sunday newspaper. Sometimes my knees would become swollen, so I'd put ice on them and relax. It felt good.

Now I see that my poor body and brain were poisoned by these "irritants" of my ordinary Sunday breakfast. My face would often swell, too—eyes, cheeks, under my chin, all puffy. I'd feel sluggish and unmotivated. But I never put this together.

Fasting Cure

It took a while to develop an awareness of all this. I realized that the only time I felt clear, focused, and full of energy was when I did a liquid fast called the Master Cleanse, which my niece Janice had discovered online. She's quite innovative at finding ways to improve her health. I always felt better fasting than I did on days that I ate. If you have any of these signs, consider that you might have food sensitivities. In terms of the Master Cleanse detox or other types of fast, please research and talk to your doctor before trying. Knowing that's supposedly how Beyoncé lost fifteen pounds shouldn't be the basis of a health decision. Really!

I distinctly remember this look on the visiting minister's face during coffee hour after the service. He was nervously trying to engage in friendly chit-chat that landed on the topic of food. "Oh, so you're not eating the delicious cake Bethany made? Here, have some!"

"I'm fasting." (I figured spiritual people would get this better than anyone).

"Oh, how long do you fast?"

Figuring I couldn't lie to a man of faith, I said, "This is the end of it today. It's been sixteen days total."

His jaw dropped. "What! You haven't had real food in sixteen days?!!"

Feeling shy and hoping he wouldn't raise his voice again, I said, "That's right, this is my longest one, and I'm almost ready for regular food. But it's okay. I feel great. I really do." There was clearly more in this conversation than he bargained for; he was just visiting our church for a day. He grabbed another piece of cake (perhaps nervous eating or thinking he could have my portion) and drifted away in the crowd. So much for dead honesty about this topic.

It was hard for years having all these sensitivities. My doctors knew I fasted and that it helped me. Sixteen days was my longest fast. It just *worked*. I felt so much better and lighter. I tried but generally didn't talk about any of this with most people. No one got the food sensitivities, even when I tried to tell them. So not surprisingly, if a family member made us a special meal that I couldn't eat parts or most of, they did not understand. Who could? "Eggs?! You can't eat eggs? They are totally natural!! They're from God."

"You can't even have a small piece of BIRTHDAY cake?! And a tiny bit of ice cream?!" "Pasta is from whole grain. That's a basic food group!"

I had to manage every social gathering trying not to be one of "those people" I feared becoming when I was growing up—the folks who had lots of allergies and went on and on and on about them. I so wanted just to be hardy.

Traveling was a nightmare since I couldn't eat most food on the plane, in snack shops, etc. Very few things were on my food plan, but eating anything else made me swell, constipated, feel mentally slow, physically gross, and emotionally depressed. After years of making mistakes by popping things into my mouth I'd later regret, giving in, and/or trying to teach myself the rules, I just ended up saying to myself: "Diane, it won't be pretty if you eat this."

Inflammation Epidemic

Saying that helped and embodied many things about the effects of eating taboo foods. Still, I felt helpless and alone dealing with these sensitivities. Then, one day while I was grocery shopping, I looked at the women and men around me in the store and realized I wasn't the only swollen person there. I saw puffy-faced and puffy-bodied people all around me. Their carts were stuffed with foods I couldn't eat—corn chips, ice cream, and bread. It occurred to me maybe they had food sensitivities too but didn't know it. It must be like an epidemic, affecting many. I felt less alone. Again, the least likely things can turn into such teachers, stones on the path to healing.

We have so much to learn about the foods we eat and about the brain and body connection. The typical processed American diet and even our toothpaste are often riddled with hidden ingredients like milk proteins and wheat fillers that inflame the body and brain. Inflammation is at the heart of all diseases—cancer, dementia, and degenerative neurological conditions.

Over the years, I have learned so much about the gut, the brain, and how I function. Increasingly we see more and more research on the significant interrelationship between the gut and digestion and how the brain is working. The symptoms of food sensitivities and brain injury can overlap a great deal, and brain injury can easily damage the gut through increased gut permeability and changes in the blood-brain barrier. There is a delicate network of communication between the gut and the brain, linking the activities of our intestines and cerebral area. A range of foods, then, can increasingly trigger an immune response in the gut.

Brain Injury and Diet

It's very important for anyone with a head injury to simplify their diet and throw out what's not working. If you have a head injury, keep a log of what you eat and how you feel. Eat whole foods, not processed ones. Limit sugar, drink lots of water, and get good exercise to keep healthy. Be good to yourself. Stock up on powerful foods like blueberries, avocado, sweet potatoes, and lots of fruits and vegetables. Use olive oil. If you have access to it, consider food sensitivity testing. You may be as surprised as I was to find out that some of your food "poisons"—e.g. asparagus—are otherwise healthy and whole, just not for you.

One book I often suggest when people know foods are bothering them but don't know where to start eliminating is J. J. Virgin's *The Virgin Diet: Lose 7 Pounds in 7 Days by Eliminating These 7 Foods*. It's an excellent book that describes what inflammation does to your body and how to eliminate the key culprits.

Here's what my diet right now has boiled down to now: lots of high-quality foods. I feel so lucky to have access to them. If you don't have access, you will need to plan carefully. More and more people are eating clean like this, which helps. I no longer have huge mood swings from foods loaded with sugar, which I hoped would be good for me but aren't, such as conventional yogurt with berries, trail mix, and protein bars. Added sugar, meaning not from the food itself as in fruit, causes body inflammation.

I no longer miss sugar (finally). I used to crave it, and it was a huge pick-me-up, but it also slammed me down. My teeth and the back of my eyes hurt from the sugar trip, and my stomach bloated. Learning that sugar bloated my gut was a game-changer. "Okay! That's over," I said to myself. I realized I could gain five pounds of water weight in a day by eating the wrong thing containing sugar. The effects of eating sugar can be hard on your sense of self, your emotional well-being. It's not just how you look. It's how you feel, too. Sugar scrapes away confidence and esteem for many people I know.

Becoming Sugar-Free

Most recently, I worked one-on-one with a nutritionist. I created a daily log of everything I put in my mouth and shared the log with her via email every day for five months. She sent me notes back daily, sort of like a report card. Little by little, I could see how different things worked. On the days I was so ravenous by dinnertime, I realized I had somehow had sugar in my breakfast or lunch. My jaw would hurt from being so tight, and I'd feel exhausted and edgy. Even many of the gluten-free muffins bloat my body—most grains do. Constipation and leg cramps come with not having enough water or movement like walking. It's not magic; it's just cause and effect. I decided I didn't need to keep rediscovering that. So, I just started skipping sugar altogether. It's on J.J. Virgin's list of inflammatory foods.

Fantastic Foods

The foods I eat now are fantastic. I can't imagine anyone seeing my meals and being anything but envious. Fruit smoothies with almond milk, coconut oil, and dates are mainstays. Lunch often includes finely chopped cauliflower that looks like rice covered with sautéed mushrooms, red peppers, and whatever other veggies we have at home. I love salsa on almost everything. Dinner might be another smoothie or stir fry, homemade soup, or an omelet. Yes, I said omelet! I can eat eggs now without my joints swelling and hurting. I am so grateful. I can travel better, too, because eggs are a protein that's almost always available.

I have an avocado every day and drink two café lattes with almond milk. Regular coffee still makes me queasy for some reason.

Neuroscientists don't disdain coffee. They actually like it. Research shows that unless it's overdone, it's good for cognitive function. I also drink decaf tea and lots of lemon water, especially first thing in the morning.

My weight is level, and while I wish I weighed a few pounds less, people say I look great. My energy is always fantastic. More recently, after the impressive research and testimonials on intermittent fasting, I have begun to learn more about that. It is said to decrease inflammation and help the brain, among other benefits. More to learn for us all. I have listed my favorite books for this mission for gut repair and healthy eating in the Notes. It's a path of many small steps and lots of learning, but totally worth it.

Chapter 13:

Learning, Learning, Learning

Mondays, Memory, and Thich Nhat Hanh

My life changed a great deal after joining Unity Temple, but that entailed more than my choir activities. It was a time of economic stress as the financial markets hit tilt in 2008, and, like the rest of the country, there were many unemployed people in the congregation.

The book I wrote in 2004, *Back in Control*, was all about the underbelly of career change and how to manage the emotional aspects of it. It talks about what people don't typically talk about with friends and family about losing a job or hating the job they have. It's the stuff people talk about with their therapist and coach — the hard stuff. I can't say I completely forgot that I wrote this book because it wasn't like I had amnesia with a blank memory. However, I just never thought about it. Ever. What's strange is that I had put my heart and soul into writing it for two years and another year into promoting it after its release. I did countless media interviews and presentations. I believed many, many people needed *Back in Control*.

Recognizing What Slid Away

After the accident, though, it was one of the things that just slid off my plate. There was one whole year, maybe longer, that I never thought about *Back in Control* once. This was an example of my brain trying its best to make everything feel normal but without the capacity to spend more energy than what it took to handle daily life and healing. One night before choir, one of the girls sitting near me said how hard it was to be between jobs. She had lost her job a couple of months earlier, and being single and self-supporting, she was concerned. She had been so kind and friendly to me from the start, a really sweet woman. I truly wanted to help her. This was real stuff. My heart felt pulled.

Later I realized something so important to me had evaporated without a trace. Talking with my choir friend initiated my reach into another world, another reality. I always thought of this book I wrote as having a mission. It was to touch people and speak to that overwhelming, depressing and self-hating space that we can slip into when we're stressed, worried about having no job—especially one that gives us a sense of purpose. I felt a silent bond as I handed her a copy of *Back in Control* before the next rehearsal began. She thanked me and put her head down. That's the other thing about that space between jobs, sometimes it has no words, and everything feels awkward. It breaks my heart that people can feel bad about losing a job during a huge economic downturn. As a coach, I saw that shame most often with people whose work ethic is very strong; those are born and bred to be contributing to the world.

Sanctuary of Monday Momentum

I started noticing that other congregation members needed career help and spoke with our minister. He consented to let me start a group called Monday Momentum. I am so grateful for his wisdom in supporting the group. It was a real shift for me in many ways.

The group met on Mondays because the first part of the week is the hardest time when you don't have a job; your friends and family are headed off to work and you're not. One of the things I always recommend for people starting career transitions is to do volunteer work. It's good for them, for others, and for the world. It's said that when you help someone else, you help yourself. This was true for me. From this Monday group, I started to see myself beyond the injury, treatment, and training—I also remembered that I am a teacher and a writer.

In the quiet of the morning, tucked away in a room inside the beautiful Frank Lloyd Wright Unity Temple, our group, ranging from five to fifteen people, gathered each Monday at nine. Each session began with a reading from works by the meditation teacher I had been on a retreat with the year before, the beloved Zen Master, Thich Nhat Hanh.

> "Aware that life is available only in the present moment and that it is possible to live happily in the here and now, I am committed to training myself to live deeply each moment of daily life. I will try not to lose myself in dispersion or be carried away by regrets about the past, worries about the future, or craving, anger, or jealousy in the present. I will practice mindful breathing to come back to what is happening in the present moment. I am determined to learn the art of mindful living by touching the wondrous, refreshing, and healing elements that are inside and around me, and by nourishing seeds of joy, peace, love, and understanding in myself, thus facilitating the work of transformation and healing in my consciousness."
>
> — **Thich Nhat Hanh**, Dwelling Happily in the Present Moment, From Interbeing: Fourteen Guidelines for Engaged Buddhism (1998) by Thich Nhat Hanh with permission of Parallax Press, www.parallax.org.

Living Deeply

I hope this passage helps you in your life as much as it still helps me. As I look back on this reading and my life now, I can see how, every day, more than once a day, it continues to guide me. Sometimes I am aware that I see the world differently than many people. I live deeply.

I'm not a Pollyanna who always sees what's positive no matter what, papering over the pain. I know the negative is there. For example, I love taking pictures to try to capture the beauty of moments, even difficult ones. Still, my practice of mindfulness is bringing myself to the present, to acknowledge what is, and to focus on the wondrous and the heroic of what's there. It feeds me and brings me out of the dream created from worrying about the past and the future. Now I realize that after having done this reading for about a year, the concepts became indelibly imprinted into my psyche. And writing this section helps me understand my own story even more. Reading the quote from Thich Nhat Hanh was a small thing that developed in the context of random events of joining a congregation, seeing a need for a group, and tapping into one of my strongest spiritual influences. This act created a steady stone under the vast water I need to walk over to create my own new life.

Everyone needs great teachers, whether they are alive and real, have passed, or are mythical. Thich Nhat Hanh is one of my greatest teachers. He's authored many books on mindfulness that have touched my life, blessing it with a deep humility and love.

During the retreat with him in 2007, I remember one Q & A session in which someone asked him about the robe he wears. He said it was maybe ten years old.

"It's a good robe and wears well. It's all I need to wear. It's enough. It's perfect." He also said he takes good care of the robe, and it takes good care of him. He also loves his Sangha (his students, nuns, and monks). He supports them as their teacher, and they support him.

I hope you can feel the same spiritual strength, vulnerability, and love I feel in this. His vulnerability is his strength. This is a different way of being than I was familiar with and not one expected of the most famous person I had ever met in my life.

The Monday Momentum group changed my life and, hopefully, the lives of the other members. Through our meetings, we made lifetime friendships. And it was so satisfying to see my writing helping and providing purpose and structure for our group members in difficult times. I asked participants to read sections from *Back in Control* between sessions and do homework to apply their learning. We discussed it all when we came back together. I saw them progress over time. Eventually, our group dwindled in size as people found new jobs and moved on.

It felt like any author's dream to see his or her book making a difference with real people. I think about how many books never even get read, let alone sit on someone's bedside to comfort them during difficult times. I still get notes and calls now and then from people who say it helped them or their adult child. That was my hope for *Back in Control* with job and life transitions, and I hope that this book will similarly offer insights and help for anyone who has suffered a concussion or wishes his or her brain would function better.

While the EMDR experience was helpful, I continued to struggle with depression like many people going through change as well as those having a brain injury. Despite the progress I had made with neurofeedback and my other treatments, I still had a belief buried deep within that nothing really makes a difference, no matter how I tried. In the end, whatever the time or investment, I told myself nothing would work out.

Thich Nhat Hanh says to hold such thoughts and feelings like a child, soothe and be with them. Little by little, I tried to use his teachings to be present and observe the struggle.

Training for Board Certification

As I continued to work toward neurofeedback board certification, I was immersed in learning. I had a list of books to read and absorb. My internships gave me pockets to put the learning into. For example, reading about EEG patterns was very challenging, but giving a brain scan is an adventure. There is a learning curve, but for me, it's much easier to *do* things than read about them. In one internship, my job entailed sitting in a dark room with patients from a hospital setting and monitoring them during the QEEG brain scans.

I felt compassion for our QEEG patients because I had been in their place. Having this same test, I'd think: "I hope my brain is okay. What if something is wrong? My poor husband's been through so much, etc." The time afterward, waiting on the results, was like no other time. You wonder, worry, and play out different life scenarios that would happen with different outcomes. Perhaps for everyone, the zone of time while waiting for medical test results is a time like no other.

Finding Heaven in EEG

I was humbled by the vulnerability of our patients in this setting and in sheer awe of being able to see "inside" their brain by watching the twenty wavy lines snaking across the screen as they breathed next to me in the dark. It was like looking into the eye of God—the brain, so complex, alive, and beautiful. Each scan was different. From the side, I could see the silhouette of the patient in refracted light from the screen. Peace, science, and God. I could have monitored scans for days. I simply loved it. I also enjoy conducting brain scans on my own patients now. People pay for these assessments, or their insurance does. But at that point in my career, if I needed to and had had the resources, I would have paid the hospital to let me sit there.

In my field, there are people who know more or less about brain scan assessment than I do. Some have other professionals do their QEEG testing and then follow directions in the reports for training their clients. It was important for me to know how to do it myself from the bottom up. I wanted to meet and breathe with patients, test many people, and see the inner workings of how training protocols are developed.

While I'd like to claim ownership of this quirky perspective, as you know from Chapter Six, I owe a debt of gratitude to my father. As a self-taught electronics buff, he spent hours and hours in our basement at night happily tinkering with electronic devices. With the QEEG brain training equipment, I see myself as my father's daughter, imprinted with a strange sense of fearlessness about my ability to learn technical things. It's in my DNA, and I am grateful for this "can learn" gift in today's world.

My learning continued. I had finished the first reading of Demos's *Getting Started in Neurofeedback* and went on to the required text by Michael Thompson, MD, and his wife, Lynda Thompson, Ph.D., called *The Neurofeedback Book*. This is a basic text in the field with lots of studies and details on the anatomy and physiology involved in neurofeedback and the conditions it treats. The book is rich but incredibly difficult for a newcomer to the field. At some points, reading it was almost comical. In one paragraph alone, I might have needed to look up four or more words because I had no idea what they were talking about. I just kept looking up words. It reminds me of Anne Lamott's famous book, *Bird by Bird*. How do you get through something tedious and immense? You do it piece by piece.

I also wanted to meet the Thompsons, these authors and pioneers of the neurofeedback field, and try to spend a little time with them.

Meeting the Masters

In the summer of 2009, almost four years after my accident, I found a way to meet the Thompsons. In my Internet wandering one night, I learned they offered a five-day workshop in Toronto a couple of times a year to help clinicians prepare for the board certification (BCIA) exam in neurofeedback. It covered the Blueprint of Knowledge in a course called "Applied Psychophysiology: Neurofeedback Combined with Biofeedback and Metacognition." What a mouthful, right?

Like Demos's workshop, it was a thirty-six-credit-hour required course for board certification with plenty of equipment and time for practicing the interventions we were reviewing. It was an international group as people came from all over the world to meet and study with these prominent authors and practitioners. It also meant spending time in the lovely Burleigh Falls at Mike and Lynda's cabin on a lake, walking in the woods, being part of a sing-along by the fire, trying bow and arrow practice, riding in canoes, and experiencing the Canadian

North. It was an amazing trip with two extraordinary leaders in the field, prolific writers, and generous, wonderful humans. I learned so much in those five days. I even started to feel like I knew something, even though their book was still hard reading for me.

The Magic of Coloring

At that point in my studies, brain physiology was still a realm I did not know as well as I needed. While complaining to my doctor about studying, she said that in medical school, she and other students had gotten these huge coloring books full of plates (pictures) of different angles and systems of the brain. I found this coloring system, which had been put together by neuroscientists Marian C. Diamond and Arnold B. Scheibels. Their system of forty-six different plates takes you through the function and structure of the brain and nervous system. It's used to train professionals like occupational therapists, physicians, and nurses. It allows you to learn it in your mind and your body. I always loved coloring and certainly respected my doctor, so I ordered it and a hundred wooden colored pencils. I spent lots of time at home and in coffee shops coloring.

As I write this, I can hardly believe I did all that coloring. But it was helpful and fascinating to learn such a complex topic on different levels. I recommend it if you want another level of absorbing information. Coloring worked like magic. If I heard a brain term that I had colored, I felt like I knew it in a different way, sort of like an old friend. "Oh yes, the nucleus accumbens region! Oh that! It's in the basal forebrain rostral part located below the corpus striatum. Plays an important role in addiction."

My brain was clearly in a much better place than a year or two before, but adding new ways of learning helped, too. I couldn't have worked through this material without adding other tools. My concentration, focus, and flexibility of thinking benefited greatly from this approach, and it helped me not to get stuck on ideas and negative moods. It's fair to say that my concentration and focus were even better than before the concussion.

Tools for Learning Impossible Amounts

Another way to deepen my learning and tamp down my sense of being overwhelmed by this detailed medical information was to take one of The Great Courses. I got a postcard in the mail from them and thought, why not? I ordered the DVDs for a thirty-six-lecture sequence called *Understanding the Brain* given by Vanderbilt University Professor Jeanette Norden, Ph.D. It covered many topics in the Blueprint of Knowledge, and listening to her talk about them with her lovely, slightly Southern accent was very informative and hugely comforting. She's a great presenter and loves science and the brain. She had many wonderful stories to illustrate concepts, including some involving her cabin on a river. I am still creeped out by an example she gave of the reptilian brain with snakes finding their way inside her cabin to seek shelter when it got cold. I just loved these DVDs and saw and/ or listened to each of them at least once. The lectures helped me feel more comfortable with the names and concepts of brain physiology.

Magical Eyes Closed Learning

That summer, I had some problems with allergies and my eyes and somehow irritated my corneas. It was hard to read for a bit, so the DVDs were perfect. Unlike reading, I could close my eyes and listen. I would also listen to a DVD before I fell asleep. This was helpful but had a surprising and quirky effect.

One morning, I was talking with a friend who was telling me her mother had recently had a stroke. I responded immediately: "Was it ischemic or hemorrhagic?"

The question just popped out of my mouth. What surprised me was that I did not know the names of these two kinds of strokes before I had gone to sleep the night before. They hadn't been part of my vocabulary. I really didn't even know the difference now that I was awake and asking my friend that question. Perhaps I would have had to go back to sleep to truly understand the difference between an ischemic and hemorrhagic stroke at that point. Overall, these Great Course lectures were first-rate and helped a lot.

By the way, an ischemic stroke involves a clot, and a hemorrhagic stroke is from a broken blood vessel hemorrhaging.

I had charts of the 16 Blueprint of Knowledge content areas and my progress covering the list of readings, and how competent I felt with each. That brought me to want to do more learning activities. I needed more direct feedback on how I was learning, so I took an online non-credit course on the Blueprint that had exams. I also purchased access to a set of practice quizzes on the content areas. At first, the quizzes went terribly, so I did them over and over again. Eventually, I wasn't sure whether I was learning those quizzes or the material itself. The online class was helpful, but the exams for it were "open book" and essay. So, I still didn't know if I could pass the three-hour exam. I especially wasn't sure if I could concentrate for that long. My life was in a state of suspension because passing the exam was going to allow me to set up shop in the right way, knowing for certain that I was thoroughly trained and credentialed to take on that responsibility. Wondering, hoping, and reading. It was hard to explain my life to most people.

Chapter 14:

Board Certification Exam— Take One!

And Then, Judy

With each step in my preparations, I interfaced with Judy Crawford, BCIA's kind and efficient executive director. She reviewed and approved my activities for meeting the application requirements for board certification. Many people take the three-hour exam after one of the thirty-six-credit hour survey classes or the Thompsons' five-day program; there is so much information, and these workshops pull it all to the front of your brain. However, the Thompsons' workshop wasn't a review for me—I had never learned most of this material before and hadn't been in clinical settings long enough to have those reference points. Reviewing materials and then taking the exam at that point would have been worthless. I needed to immerse myself in the information, really learn it, and then review it.

I was also worried about not sleeping well at a training away from home and then the test setting being noisy, cold, or otherwise distracting. These environmental considerations sound minor, but if you've spent hundreds of hours preparing for an exam, it's wise to optimize the environmental factors to do your best.

Later in the preparation game, I found out I could take the BCIA exam administered by a proctor at my neighborhood library, also saving me time and travel expenses. I started to feel like I needed more information about the exam. After studying in different ways for almost two years, I figured I should try to use the test itself to get a sense of it. Judy reminded me I could take it over if needed.

Finally, Test Day

I set a time and arranged for a proctor. It was at two on a Thursday afternoon on November 11, 2010—just about a month and five years after the accident that changed my world. I met the proctor at the library at the end of my block and settled in for the long haul. The room was quiet, and although I hadn't slept well the night before, it still was in the comfort of my own bed.

The exam was vexing. The items went a step further than my study and review. I had to use my knowledge to make inferences to get answers. The questions weren't straightforward like, "What's the frequency of waves referred to as High Beta?" with four responses to choose from. They were more like, "Given the change in frequency of brain waves likely to occur with cocaine use, what's the best protocol with neurofeedback to reduce cravings?"

The exam shattered me. It was so much harder than I ever expected, despite how diligently I had prepared. Even though I knew I could take it again, this had been my one project since the accident in 2005. It was my love, my focus, and my passion, and I just wanted it to go well. I wanted to feel that if I worked hard, something good would happen. And it was clear I had learned so, so much both in workshops and studying on my own.

I started to mull over how I had studied for this exam. For my state licensing exam to become a therapist, I had formed a study group of friends. We had all learned together, divided up the required reading list, and then taught and quizzed each other about what we had read. Here, I had been studying alone, coloring alone in coffee shops, and although I had loved every second of it, I knew mine was a nontraditional path. It was something that grew out of my own need to heal from an injury that had turned my life upside down. I knew Elsa would be in my corner no matter what. I had no idea how old she was, but she got her Ph.D. in her fifties. I slugged out the exam for the whole three hours, struggling with questions in a way that you'd never guess how much I studied.

It wasn't until after the exam was over that I could see how much of myself I had put into it. What it meant to prepare on my own, to take my study cards on every vacation, listen to my DVDs, organize the information into my own "Cliff notes" cheat sheets, and summarize my cheat sheets into smaller summaries, hoping that handling the information so much would help it sink in. All the people from the field I'd met, all the trips I'd taken to pursue this dream. It was a lot.

As the autumn leaves crunched under my feet, I walked north on our block from the library to my condo, my head thick and tired. I knew I had failed the exam. It'll be best to take a break before I started studying again, I told myself. I'd start back in a week. One week, then back on the horse. Plans always help me. I could do this . . . just needed to take a rest first.

The Dragon Show

When I walked in the door, my husband asked how I did. I told him it went horribly and then sat down across from him in our living room. I didn't have much else to say. I didn't know what to do besides think about when I'd start studying again. I felt like the wind had been knocked out of me, but I was moving slowly, trying to catch my breath, hoping I wouldn't deeply disappoint my husband, who had invested right along with me. I had taken time away from our lives, and we'd spent money on these trips. My heart was heavy. I knew he would try not to be disappointed, but how could he not be? My quest had consumed our lives for almost two years.

Deep negative thinking began inside my newly healed brain. The dragons of my darkest inner thoughts began to creep in. Whatever made me think I could teach myself advanced brain physiology and neurofeedback systems outside of a university, a teaching center? I am in my fifties and had a head injury. This is something for "them"—other people luckier than me. Perhaps it was like trying to teach myself nuclear physics from library books or TED talks. Not to be done. I'd worked hard, but it wasn't enough this time. There was a right way to learn, and I wasn't in on it. I don't belong in this field, with these people.

A few hours later, our home phone rang, interrupting this storm in my head. It was Judy Crawford, which confused me because I'd never talked to her on our home phone. I knew she'd feel bad for me, and I would find that unbearable. As we started to talk, she spoke very slowly.

"Is this Diane Wilson?" (I knew she knew it was me. I couldn't figure out why she was doing it and talking so slowly. I figured this conversation was hard for her.)

"Yes. This is Diane."

"Diane Grimard Wilson?"

"Yes." *Maybe it's not Judy*, I thought. Feeling defeated, I sighed. I certainly wasn't up for some stupid, random sales call on top of everything.

"This is Judy Crawford from the Board Certification International Alliance." Her slow, measured pace didn't sound like her at all.

"I know," I said, rushing my words. "I'll take it again. Or just let me know when this will be scored. I know I can take it again." Bad news is hard to give, I figured. I tried to make it easier for her. I felt sure that what she had to tell me was difficult, knowing I had done all the steps and more with such diligence.

"Are you sitting down?"

Please don't make this any harder, Judy.

"Yes?"

"I wanted you to know I was able to score your exam myself this afternoon. The proctor faxed your sheet to us. I know you wanted to know. Are you sitting down?" *Judy, this is making it harder, and don't worry, I got the news. It's okay.* I was on the verge of crying now.

"Yes, I'm sitting down." Across the living room, my husband sat frozen with his eyes opened wide. It still didn't sound like Judy because she was talking so slowly and deliberately.

"Your score was an 84." I knew it. It was too low to pass. An 84! *Okay, okay!... I got it. I know I didn't pass.*

"It was an 84!" she said again, loudly.

"Okay." Totally confused, I thought, *why is she doing this?*

"That means you scored in the top tier of anyone who has ever taken the exam."

"WHAT?"

OMG! That group included neuropsychologists, graduate students, and medical doctors. *OMG! Was this real?*

I was stunned. My husband looked stunned too, but he still didn't know why. I asked her a couple of questions, and she started to sound like the person I knew. She was at least as happy as I was. With tears rolling down my face, my husband began to understand and cry, too. He'd gotten the news!

"You did it! You did better than most people who take the test!" She sounded truly shocked herself and said she was surprised and wanted me to know right away. Her voice still sounded excited, but it became more normal as we talked. I realized she was stunned herself and couldn't wait to deliver the news.

"I called on your home phone because I thought since it's late, I could definitely reach you there."

I sighed. "Yes, I am at home. I'm tired and was just planning when I'd start studying again."

In a collage of elation and information, I expressed my huge appreciation to Judy. I offered my kindest thanks to her for answering all my questions over the last two years. I hadn't known anyone else who was preparing and taking the exam when I was. My Chicago colleagues had taken it years before, and people I met in the workshops already worked in the field or were in school and took the exam shortly after the workshop.

I don't think I had ever seen my husband happier than in that moment. We did a loud happy dance, jumping up and down with him saying, "Hon, you did it!" over and over.

My husband wanted to share the news during our next church service's "Joys and Sorrows." I stood next to him in front of our congregation. The whole thing made me super emotional. My face was beet red; I was frozen, smiling with tears trickling onto my cheeks. I was glad he was the one to share it. Our congregation cheered, and after the service, people were so congratulatory. It was truly a moment of triumph for me. It was me, coming up against the world, being run over, finding support, and conquering big obstacles—me with a lot of help.

In my life since the injury, part of me had hidden in the shadows of myself. Once I realized I was injured, I felt damaged, disabled, and less-than. But I never knew I felt that was so much in trying to be okay and wanting so much to be okay. I really didn't know I felt so damaged by what had happened to me. I had a sense of not feeling strong, of not wanting to be social, or knowing what to say or do. After all, something so big had happened to me, and I figured most people probably didn't or wouldn't understand, especially at that point when knowledge on brain trauma and its impact on people's lives was lacking, as it still is for many.

After passing the exam, I no longer felt damaged. I was finally okay again. And knowing I had done something very difficult, and done it very well, helped.

Chapter 15:

Life Continues: Milestones and Then the Unthinkable

Many things happened after passing the board certification exam in November 2010, and much of it was good. My recovery from the concussion, post-concussion syndrome, and brain trauma was complete. I had learned ways to manage life with food intolerances and soften their impact.

Overall, now, I'm more sensitive to my brain and how it's functioning than most people. I know how my injury can impact me as time goes on with early dementia and cognitive decline. I take good care of my brain. The prize of this crazy journey is that I now use every single step of it in my work with my clients. Working with neurofeedback is my passion; I can't imagine my life without it. We are doing some amazing things in this field of applied neuroscience that I want you to know about and benefit from, even if you've never had a head bump, concussion, or ADD. These insights and tools will help you become a better version of you no matter what your situation is. First, let's bring you up to date on some of the major milestones I hit along the way.

The Legal Case

In October 2007, almost two years after the accident, I filed a lawsuit to recover the costs of my medical treatment from the insurance company of the fellow who ran into me. The court deposition I described in Chapter Eleven was a year later. Then, not having reached a settlement, we moved toward a trial in the fall of 2009. My husband and I met with the lawyer, our chatty, personable, sports-loving, straight-talking lawyer. He's a member of our community, coached a kids' sports team, and seems to know everyone in the area. *Although he remembers this differently,* what I came away from that meeting with was the understanding that if I cried during the trial, the case would be thrown out. That means there would be no chance of any settlement.

Crying was a major issue for me.[5] Even after close to ten sessions of EMDR, I couldn't talk about the accident and being injured without tears running down my face or, at a minimum, choking up. Yes, part of me did not want to know or acknowledge how the accident significantly impacted my brain and life. However, there was another part of me that did know it. And that part, equally out of my grasp, was very sad about the loss of time, momentum on my career, cognitive function, and having a secret I could not easily claim. To this day, my voice often chokes, and I feel a flood of emotion when talking about having had a brain injury. It just happens. I can't help it.

While disappointed, my husband and I opted out of a trial after our lawyer's briefing because it promised to be as traumatic as my initial injury. The legal case for my accident settled out of court, and when outstanding medical fees were paid, the remaining payment for me was less than $1,000. There was basically no compensation for the time entailed or trauma I'd endured. Next to nothing.

I felt devastated and somehow ashamed. It wasn't that I was looking for some big settlement, but I was disappointed that the legal system somehow would come to depict my experience, the two years of ongoing neuropsychological treatment with Dr. Elsa Baehr, an esteemed clinical psychologist in her field, as somehow not the kind of injury one would be compensated for. My time, pain, and suffering

---

5   In writing this book, I contacted our attorney, our friend, who said this was a misunderstanding and that neither he nor the judge had said that if I cried the case would be thrown out. Our recall of this conversation is different. I can't explain these differences and have moved on from it.

didn't figure in the financial settlement. I was ashamed since I felt I was being told how I recovered, the length of time it took, and how much care I needed were all my fault. Knowing what I know now of concussion and the path to recovery, I feel vindicated but believe my settlement was unfair.

I am certain I am not alone in being impacted by the limited or nonexistent understanding of concussion and post-concussive symptoms. Many people have suffered from brain injuries and much more than I have. Query into the impact of concussions on brain function and health began in earnest in 2005. That's when forensic pathologist Dr. Bennet Omalu autopsied the beloved retired football player Mike Webster and discovered advanced brain deterioration. Webster had suffered terrible headaches, mood swings, depression, and cognitive decline. A retired football hero, at the point of his death, he lived in his car and suffered wrenching physical pain. He was estranged from his family, who worried so much about him but hardly recognized the often-raging man he had become. The syndrome Omalu coined to describe Webster's battered brain was chronic traumatic encephalopathy (CTE). Mike Webster's brain pathology had emerged, and it flourished in the years after retiring from the National Football League.

Omalu's work was first published in 2005 in the scientific journal *Neurosurgery*. However, the full impact of concussion on the brain was years away from being recognized, especially in the nonscientific communities. My moderate concussion was not close to the long-term repetitive damage that professional football players endure. But research is consistently emerging about how brain pathology can occur with far less physical trauma. For example, high school football players show pathological brain patterns from many fewer hits overall in their lives. Enduring brain trauma can occur in players who were never diagnosed with a concussion or incurred as many hard hits as Webster. Those playing other sports are impacted as well. We have just begun to understand the brain, how it's injured, what it means to be injured, and how it heals.

There are two things I am grateful for in handling the settlement: First, I never lived my life hating or resenting the person who drove into me. I never spent time or mental energy that way. It was an accident. I have made many mistakes in my life, and accidents do happen. I don't know this person. I doubt I will ever meet him again. His behavior impacted my life, but it wasn't directed at me personally. I have met people who deeply resented others for years for much lesser offenses. I dodged an emotional pothole on this one. My teacher Thich Nhat Hanh would be proud of me.

Second, I never proceeded with the hope or expectation of some huge financial compensation for what the accident took from me. It wasn't something I thought about. I've worked with clients who had a potential financial settlement in the picture and often felt it compromised their ability to get well. Thinking like that could have compromised my healing and elongated the process. You could easily argue that the anosognosia, where my brain opted out of me acknowledging my injury, also kept me from resenting the driver and hoping for some settlement. I would say, fair enough. However, even now, years later, I still feel the same. I don't think about or resent the driver or spend time longing for a more equitable restitution. I am grateful for all my teachers and training which has allowed this to be the case. My life is mine. This is my wish for everyone.

My husband and I do not live in the past any more than necessary. We don't mull this over and over. I don't think the settlement was fair, but I have had to focus on my life going forward. That made for a better life during the recovery and reconstruction when I've needed my resources. Finances can make life easier; I truly appreciate that more and more as I get older. I hope with more understanding and recognition of what brain trauma is and does, others will find it easier to get compensation for these life-changing injuries.

New Tribes

Many milestones served to widen my network with some fascinating people. While I had a world of people who didn't know or understand what I had gone through—not that I was very helpful in sharing that—I was also developing some new tribes. I had researched and purchased my own brain scan equipment and taken an intensive, advanced training in giving QEEG scans. The equipment was expensive (think the price of a new car), and I recall the joy of sending in the very last payment for it. With the equipment came the opportunity to join and become active in ongoing learning circles. Currently, I attend the case reviews and practice circles hosted by NewMind Technologies, a leader in QEEG software with Dr. Richard Soutar and his colleague Rob Longo, as well as training by Brainmaster Technologies with Tom Collura and his team. Another group I joined after becoming officially a colleague and not a patient is called EEG Chicago, a group of board-certified neurofeedback clinicians from the Chicago area, including Dr. Kathy Abbott. Overall, unless I'm deeply immersed in writing, I'm actively involved in networking and information sharing with them and others in my field. They are a generous network of colleagues and friends. I learn from everyone and belong to many tribes of excellent people in this phase of my life.

I still talk with Elsa on occasion. She continues to work, albeit on a reduced schedule at an age when most people would have retired decades earlier. She's still sharp, witty, kind, and has great humor. I called her yesterday, but she couldn't talk because she was in her singing lesson.

New Training Tools

My life involves daily learning about this new field I am in and have come to love. I continue to monitor changes and improvements in brain training devices and practices and incorporate them into my practice, where appropriate. As a baby boomer, I am quite motivated to keep my brain healthy and sharp as aging threatens to take its toll.

One brain training tool I've invested in, become certified on, and found quite impressive is the Interactive Metronome (IM). It's behaviorally based brain training that one of my clients refers to as "the slapping and clapping." It involves syncing body movements (generally clapping) with an audio rhythm. It improves neuro-timing, which is basic to how the brain and body work.

I started using the IM program intensively on myself after a friend pointed out he believed he processed information faster than I did. That, by the way, was like waving a red flag in front of a bull. After working so hard on my recovery, I am proud of how my brain works. It's like I have superpowers, especially my memory. I feel like: "I have a great brain!"

The IM helps memory, information processing speed, and speech fluency, plus my ability to come in more precisely on the musical beat in choir. It's a great peak performance tool for athletes, performers, and executives, and it also helps treat Parkinson's, dementia, and ADD. It's also nice for brain brightening in executives with very competitive jobs who always need to be sharp, on their toes. Many people feel sharper after the first session and a little worn out from the clapping. A typical program is ten to fifteen sessions, occurring two to three times per week.

New Trials

Another important milestone is writing. Since I joined Unity Temple in 2008 and started to think about writing again, like with many things, I had a collage of feelings about it.

On the one hand, I have always believed I was meant to be a writer. I work hard at coaching and counseling, which are my passions, but writing is my purpose. There may be better writers than me, I know that, but it feels like my job here. It was sewn into my shirt by God or whoever does that task at some very early point in life. From my earliest vision, I wanted to find topics people needed to hear about and then touch, inform, support, and inspire them when they felt as lonely and lost as I have felt at times. I wanted to help families learn and find compassion for what they each might be experiencing. In the same way some people imagine growing up, marrying, and having a white picket fence, I had always hoped to write at least three books in my life.

On the other hand, the brain injury was a vexing event because my very being, the most basic sense of who I am, my motivations and needs were involved in the disorganization. Without realizing it until recently, I had started to write this book several times since 2009. Every writing class or retreat brought me back to the story of my injury. During every situation in which I had a deep writing moment, the story surfaced.

To begin writing this manuscript, I spent eight weeks going through my journals from over the ten years post-injury to understand, gather content, and prepare. I had so many files tucked away titled New Book, Book 2011, or BOOK that all started with my car accident. It's evidence of how fragmented I was; I never realized how many times I had started and would then, later, begin anew.

Maybe subconsciously, it showed I wasn't sure I believed I could write another book. Instead, I wondered if I would be destined to stare into the bakery case desperately wanting something that I couldn't have, like one of those people who always wants to write a book but never does.

Could I really put this all together and tell this story?

Would anyone want to hear it?

I wasn't sure. I am grateful to my husband, who answered this question countless times with a definitive YES.

And he helped me along the way, validating my experience when I said, "OMG, this IS what happened, isn't it?"

He made comments like, "That's exactly what happened. How could you remember it so precisely?" Yet, I still wonder how I could ever forget some of this.

On Writing and Careers

In the world of career coaching, there is a focus on helping individuals learn about themselves and their gifts to find their true calling. The goal is to select a job or work environment that features our genius so that we will be in sync with our true selves.

That's all very good, but Thich Nhat Hanh and others talk about letting your calling find you. We need to understand our gifts or strengths and then look outside ourselves to see what the world needs and align our energy with that. That creates a powerful synergy. My calling took me here. Often, I feel the gravity of sitting and marinating in my fears, but I also truly believe the world needs more stories about the brain, concussion, neurofeedback, food, the gut, and music and the nontraditional paths to find our way back to who we really are. But, for the record, I believe the world needs your story,

The Unthinkable

Since starting this book, with the music director's permission, I have stepped back now and then from the life-giving joy of being in the choir to focus on this project. In March of 2018, I returned to sing in a major piece we were presenting, Fauré's *Requiem*. At Unity Temple, a friend had dashed upstairs in our newly renovated music library to get me a musical score. I hadn't been on the second level since this historic Frank Lloyd Wright gem had reopened after an extensive renovation. I bounced up the stairs behind him. Excited to be back, I was talking with him and turned my head. I was looking at the renovation and walked straight into a thick glass window I hadn't seen. The glass didn't break, but within minutes two goose eggs sprouted on my head. I felt hot and dizzy, and my forehead was numb. I knew I had a concussion. Sure enough, that same night during choir practice, old recognizable symptoms came back—that overwhelmed with a headachy feeling, hurting eyes, exhausted at the end of the day, challenging speech and processing, nausea, and my balance was off. I thought, *Why this? Why now?*

But it's helped as I have been writing about my journey. It's offered a miniature version of the original concussion, which I had felt so inarticulate in trying to describe at that time. This recent injury was a "slight concussion," and my first was "moderate." Have you ever seen the Prudential Building in New York City? It's massive and pointed at the top. From one of my Chicago architectural boat tours, I learned that Chicago has its own Prudential Building, which some call Pru2. It's the same distinctive building only in miniature, meaning the same size as an ordinary skyscraper. That's the image my concussion always brings up when I try to explain the difference—a miniature but still big duplicate with all the essential elements. "This is my Pru2."[6]

---

6   For accuracy: I mentioned this analogy recently to a choir member, Ed McDevitt, who is an art and architectural expert. He said it is technically not accurate since Pru 2 is a building in Chicago that doesn't look like the Prudential Building in New York City. While the analogy doesn't work perfectly, the concept still works of something small compared to its duplicate that is much larger.

Chapter 16:

Lessons on Concussion

So, thirteen years after my accident, confident that my brain was finally put back in great working order, I was devastated to hurt my head again. Embarrassed, even though no one saw my head bounce off the thick glass window that I thought was an open door, I took my seat in the second row of the soprano section in the huge, semi-circle facing our choir director. My face and ears started to burn, feeling flush and red hot. My head felt like a bursting tomato. A friend sitting next to me asked if I was okay and offered to get some ice; I nodded yes. I felt a little dizzy, and I wanted it all just to go away. I started feeling nauseous, and like I should leave. However, I didn't want to walk the four blocks home in the dark alone, not knowing how I'd feel once I stood up. I usually walk home with another choir member, my neighbor, who is a singer as well as a physician—not that the last part usually matters.

I don't remember getting home that night. But I do remember being home, lying on the couch with an ice pack on my forehead, and noticing the look on my husband's face. I imagine him thinking: "My wife just went back to choir and got a head injury while finally getting to write a book about her concussion journey." My own poor brain was stuck: "This isn't happening. This can't happen. I don't want this to happen. No!" My beloved Dr. Locke had retired two months earlier. I missed her so much already. We called the new doctor the first thing in the morning.

Herein lies the wisdom of life: everything gives us something we can use, right? This accident truly has given me a second chance.

It's a chance to share lessons about concussion, some of it informed by significant advances made in the field of concussion treatment and my hard-won insights since my first concussion journey that I now could articulate much better. I hope you will not have to learn these lessons on your own. My wish is that these insights and resources will equip you for the unexpected, which, we all know, we can expect.

Your Injury and Diagnosis May Unfold

Be aware that however you feel in the first moments after head trauma, whether it's from an auto accident, a head bump, a blast, or sports injury, may not be how you will feel the next day or a few days later. Based on my first concussion, that was clear. The morning after was much more difficult than the day of the accident when I was also probably in shock. From being jolted, the brain may develop bruising and swelling over time, causing other symptoms, which also will manifest over time. If, for instance, you hurt your leg, the bruise seldom shows up immediately. Same with broken blood vessels and brain swelling. Headaches can occur, and other symptoms can cascade. Getting the "all clear" right away from an ER or even your primary care doctor may not be the most accurate diagnosis. After this recent head bump, it was clear right away I probably had a concussion.

Hopefully, most doctors these days are more concussion aware than ever. But I still hear people say they didn't follow up after an accident since an ER doctor didn't tell them to, and they don't want to be a "baby." We can't assess ourselves very well in these situations. As patients, we may not accurately report how we feel to health care professionals—or people close to us—and even when we do, our judgment may be impaired. Also, the doctor may have told us to seek follow-up, but we weren't capable of processing or remembering this information at the time. Tricky stuff, huh?

See a Doctor. Don't Delay

Research supports that the sooner you are treated for brain trauma, the better your outcomes will be. Ask your primary care (PC) doctor for a referral to a specialist in concussions. While my primary care physician Dr. Locke did well at the time of the first concussion, I found it much easier to get more resources that were appropriate for me this time around.

Diane Roberts Stoler and Barbara Albers Hill wrote a comprehensive book called *Coping with Concussion and Mild Traumatic Brain Injury*. It's excellent and provides many practical insights about brain injury and recovery, including a list of questions to ask prospective practitioners, such as:

— How many concussion cases have they treated?

— What percentage of the provider's practice is related to concussion?

— Have they attended any conferences or courses in the last two years on concussion?

Since our judgment can be impaired when injured, Stoler and Hill also suggest having another person who is objective help us choose a provider.

Our understanding of neurophysiology and brain trauma are constantly growing. Having the most current thought from experts in the field is to your advantage. In the case of my second concussion, my primary care doctor suggested seeing an ophthalmologist since I had eye pain, and the goose eggs I had were above my right eye.

I wasn't convinced an ophthalmologist was the best professional for me but took the referral to a doctor at Loyola University's Maywood Park campus in the western suburb of Chicago. It's one of Chicago's major teaching hospital systems, and there I saw Dr. Eileen Gable.

Once I met her, I realized I had hit the jackpot. A distinguished senior clinician, she is kind, soft-spoken, asked me many questions, listened very carefully, performed the basic neurological tests, and then examined my sore eye. I felt she understood me and my concerns. Of course, as luck would have it, by the time I was sitting directly in front of the good doctor, the goose eggs on my forehead were almost completely gone. They had disappeared during the second night after the bump. With her ophthalmoscope in hand, she leaned into my face and peered deeply into my eye, behind and above it. She said it was irritated but not damaged. She explained the pros and cons of getting a CT scan (computerized tomography), and I voted against it unless it was necessary. A CT scan's radiation exposure is equivalent to that of two hundred X-rays. After reading Dr. Keith Black's book *Brain Surgeon*, I vowed never to get X-rays unless I absolutely needed them. Dr. Black says he never even gets dental X-rays.

The swelling was inside above my eye socket, and that was creating the pain. Most fortunate though, she had just returned from a conference on concussion and was able to share the most current thought and research on rehabilitation. These were her recommendations for my diagnosis of "slight concussion."

Consider Omega 3

Dr. Gable prescribed a protocol of massive doses of high-grade Omega-3s, specifically, fish oil from wild-caught sources. "It will make a huge difference. Your brain is made of oil, and bathing it in high-quality oils as it heals will make a dramatic difference in healing time."

My husband and I went to Whole Foods supermarket on the way home. For the first two weeks, I took several times the normal dosage of Omega-3 spread throughout the day. Check with your doctor to determine the exact dosage. It was a lot, but I did it, and it helped me significantly to feel and function better. After two weeks, I tapered down some but still took a very high dosage. Even now, over a year and a half later, I am religious about taking fish oil. As an almost-vegetarian, I first wanted to look for plant-based sources like nuts for Omega-3. However, coming home from my appointment, I decided just to do what the doctor ordered. Some professionals say plant-based Omega-3s can provide the same essentials.

As with all my suggestions, of course, talk with your doctor before beginning a regimen. Fish oil contains essential ingredients the human body cannot make but needs. It is extremely important to your body and brain. The Omega-3 fatty acids support many body systems. People who have fish and shellfish allergies should avoid this, as well as those with certain heart and blood conditions.

Cod liver oil was considered a cure-all (and a punishment) by many parents when I was growing up. Kids were made to swallow the oil when they misbehaved. Maybe that's because cod liver oil helps the brain and body in so many ways. Maybe it helps us be and do our best after taking it. Cod liver oil is a type of fish oil but has the advantage of increased amounts of EPA and DHA, vitamins A and D, and hence, has a powerful anti-inflammatory effect on the body and may also reduce anxiety and feelings of depression. I took it for a while and felt like I was doing the right thing for myself. I recommend the lemon-flavored liquid version.

"Be Careful with the Screens"

Dr. Gable advised staying away from my computer, iPad, and phone screens for a couple of days, at least, and then easing back into them. The brain is stressed by concentrating on a screen, and the blue light wavelengths from digital screens suppress the hormone melatonin that helps induce sleep at night. The brain needs deep rest to repair itself.

I believe the blue light exposure from our screens will be like cigarette smoke in the 1950s. We're surrounded by it but don't realize its impact on us. Just for the record, I am wearing my blue-blocking amber-tinted glasses as I write this. Especially at night, I like to reduce the stress on my eyes and brain and, of course, get great sleep.

My friend, nurse Lynn Lennon, neurofeedback and nutritional expert, describes it best: "Screens present multiple challenges for the eyes and brains. The blue spectra that is predominant in most modern screen-based electronics is particularly not a friend of mitochondria. Mitochondria do not like that particular nanometer of light, especially when it is a tonic (steady) signal."

Mitochondria are the cell's powerhouses, and they create energy, mediate growth, and signal activities. www.britannica.com/science/mitochondrion

Ms. Lennon points out that screens give off a flicker rate our unconscious is stimulated by, even if our conscious mind deletes this very brief activity. The fast flicker rates of screens, as well as fluorescent lights, make the brain work harder. She notes: "The sun doesn't flicker, thankfully!"

"Get Adequate Sleep"

Doctor's orders. This is not the time to skimp on sleep. Because the injured brain uses more energy during the day to function and to repair itself, I felt exhausted by the end of the afternoon, once I went back to work. Some people believe that you should stay awake immediately after a concussion injury, that falling asleep is dangerous. Dr. Alice Alexander from University of Arkansas Medical Sciences states,

"If the person who is injured is awake and holding a conversation, you can let him or her fall asleep as long as they are not developing any other symptoms such as dilated pupils or issues with walking. Usually after a concussion, a person may be dazed or may vomit," explains Dr. Alexander. "For children, we advise parents to wake up the child a couple of times during the night to make sure they can be aroused."

Dr. Alexander states:

> "Unless a doctor says the person needs further treatment, the injured person should sleep and rest."

"Get Physical Exercise"

The ophthalmologist, Dr. Gable, suggested resting a couple of days but not stopping aerobic exercise completely since it keeps the body systems working. Instead, she advised reducing intensity and duration with gentle to moderate cardiovascular activity and recommended walking. The thought was that hitting the sofa and taking lots of time away from normal responsibilities may not be helpful. That included work.

I saw her on a Friday and had the weekend to take it easy. But she was clear that I should go back to the office the next week even if I had to make my days shorter. Gulp. I told her what my work was like, and she said there was no reason to stay home. Okay...

"Eat Whole Unprocessed Foods"

I was surprised when the ophthalmologist Dr. Gable also suggested I should watch my diet. She's an eye doctor but then, still a doctor. Her advice was to eat food, real basic foods, and eliminate ones without nutritional value like potato chips. And watch the sugar. The trauma floods the brain with inflammation. Processed foods contain fillers, colorings, and preservatives that are believed to, or do, cause inflammation. Eating processed foods and/or ones with added sugar will increase our level of inflammation, move us away from recovery and result in us feeling poorly. I was grateful for the new ideas and reminders of things I knew but just wasn't remembering in those moments. Dr. Gable was very helpful overall and said I didn't need to see her again unless I had problems with my eye.

Share Your Story

At the time of the 2005 concussion, I had no understanding or language for talking about my symptoms. Much of what I went through, I couldn't or wouldn't talk about with other people. These days, there is more openness and conversation about head injury and concussion. People are more receptive to the topic. This time around, I told my clients and friends about my concussion and the effect on my speech and organizational skills and that I also was feeling a little overwhelmed. Everyone was sympathetic. I generally felt okay, and after taking a couple of days to rest and taking massive amounts of Omega-3s, I could work and be present. I just wasn't at the top of my game. My cognitive processing lag was clear to my clients and me. I always want to model self-care, work, and progress, so I strived to address my challenges openly. I said things like this: "Give me another second here to set this training up. Things are moving a little slower today."

It's real. Accidents and head injuries happen. I now know how to take care of myself and when to get help.

And there is healing power in sharing your life with a receptive audience—like you, my readers, here. But in some situations, it won't feel right. In some jobs, sharing might not be accepted well, but in most places, communicating about your injury will explain any challenges or changes in your performance and hopefully result in your employer giving you a little slack as you do your best while your brain heals. For some, traumatic brain injury may be covered by the protections of the Americans with Disabilities Act (ADA) and afford you special accommodations at work, if needed. To determine if your concussion would meet the criteria, contact www.eeoc.gov. Being able to share in-depth about your injury and how it happened can deactivate the emotional triggers. If your friends and family can't hear this kind of information about you, look for a group of brain trauma survivors to meet with either in person or online. Social media is bursting with resources and ways to connect with others with brain trauma. Stoler and Hill's book is rich with resources, and I list some in Appendix 1. Bottom line: it's harder to heal in isolation, and there is much to learn about brain injury and concussion.

Everyone's Journey Will Be Different

As we try to understand ourselves, or friends and family try to understand us, after a concussion or other brain trauma, we may want to compare ourselves to see if we're doing this right. It's natural. You may want to compare your concussion at age eight to one now or to some sports figure's injury. But everyone's recovery is different. There are many factors in how people react and heal—their health, prior history, their age at the time of the injury, are among the many factors. Younger kids are likely to heal much faster than aging adults. Research shows that among adults, age (older is more likely) and gender (being female) are significant factors in the likelihood of being treated for post-concussive symptoms.

Other factors may include environmental stress that's taking away from your healing energy. Previous history may be powerful and laden with psychological implications. I grew up in a family where people got a "knock in the head" for "acting up," and physical punishment was not questioned. It was the standard. I sometimes wonder if that history affected me in a way that created the anosognosia. My brain did NOT want to, or feel safe, acknowledging that it was injured even to myself. "I am okay. I will be okay."

Address Your Fears

A week after my second concussion, I visited my very sick friend Trish at Northwestern Memorial Hospital in downtown Chicago. At that time, my eye was still hurting a lot. I was thinking maybe I did need a CT scan and had made the wrong decision turning it down at Loyola. Seeing her lying in a hospital bed, getting in touch with my own health, and noting I was literally in a hospital, I went to their emergency room for a CT scan referral. Without pause, they screened me for "needs nothing immediately" but gave me a referral to their Concussion Clinic, where I was seen the next morning. They were great: efficient, kind, and deliberate.

While thirteen years before, I couldn't even get an appointment with a neurologist, this time, I was seen by one very present neurologist and a team of distinguished professionals and lanky young interns at Northwestern's Concussion Clinic. It was the day after my ER visit. Led by a distinguished doctor, who was an excellent listener, the team performed a series of neurological tests and gave me a thumbs up for the progress of my recovery. Besides, it was still early; the eye pain, fatigue, slight confusion, and forgetfulness were to be "expected" for about ten days after the injury. They said I could come back if I needed anything. As I looked into the eyes of this kind but deliberate doctor, I believed he understood my situation. I was not "brushed off," and I knew they would help if my symptoms worsened. I was okay. And, upon leaving, my eye pain stopped. Listen to your inner voice and address your fears the best ways you can. Stress and uncertainty make everything worse.

Expect Ups and Downs

Even though my days were shorter, and I felt super tired at night, I knew my healing would be a process. Over time, there were days when I felt like my old self. I was relieved the Omega-3s and all the other things I was doing were making a difference. I believed I'd dodged a bullet, and this would be an easier recovery than before.

Then, I had a couple of big deadlines at work come together at once—a corporate coaching proposal and a big insurance report. It was humbling. All my old symptoms seemed to come back, and I felt trapped in a body that didn't work well. Plus, there was nothing I could do. My speech felt slow. Words flew away before I caught them to finish sentences. I would be explaining something to someone and suddenly stop... since the words just didn't happen. It's embarrassing to be looking directly at someone in a conversation and have this occur. In writing, I struggled to string the words and thoughts together to share concepts. Connections and overarching themes became hard to synthesize. This was my prefrontal cortex going offline—the brain's supervisor in charge of the executive functions. I felt powerless, as if all my efforts to proceed as though all was well were in vain. I didn't feel near my best.

It had been four months since I ran into the thick glass window. Northwestern Concussion Clinic said I could come back if there were problems, but they also said my deficits appeared subtle. When you're self-employed and work one-on-one with people, no communication deficit feels subtle. It felt noticeable that I was more easily confused about appointment times and scheduling. Still, I could do my job. Overall, I expected things could go up and down, but I felt like I was suddenly going backward.

Recognize This Might Not Be a Quick Fix

Head injuries can affect you for months, even a year or more afterward. Don't be discouraged if you have flare-ups and symptoms, especially under stress. Our brain must work harder under stress. It's important to stay with all your strategies for managing stress to help you and your brain—backing off on things and saying "no" when needed to make your plate manageable, and to help you feel more in control. Don't let yourself forget you are still recovering, even if your mind wants to forget and just "be okay." You'll make better choices that way. Your recovery doesn't have to last forever, especially with good self-care.

Learn About Concussion and Post-Concussion Symptoms

It was only in writing this book that I have realized the wide range of possible symptoms that can result from head trauma. Again, Stoler and Hill's book is an excellent source for understanding the scope of how head trauma can impact us. They group symptoms into four types of difficulties we may experience. These include:

1. **Physical** (fatigue, light sensitivity, sleep disturbances, and headaches)
2. **Mental** (attention, memory, and speech)
3. **Emotional** (fear of "going crazy," depression, mood swings, PTSD, substance addiction)
4. **Behavioral patterns:** (Fearful, confrontational demeanor, temper explosion, impatience)

Take time to learn more about these signs and symptoms from the experts and teach those around you about potential challenges in these areas. All this will help you understand your life and take more effective control of your recovery and treatment.

Log and Increase Self-Awareness

Keep a log of how you feel for a couple of weeks or longer—at the very least during the first week—to help you keep track of your behavior. If writing it down seems tedious, consider making an audio log. Note your mood, activities, and diet. That way, you are more likely to see any patterns you might not appreciate in the moment or think to tell your health care provider. Keeping a journal can be an incredibly valuable tool overall.

Pull in Tools: You May Need Several

Four months after my second concussion, I called my brilliant neurofeedback colleague Corey Feinberg. He was trained in Dr. Elsa Baehr's lab and worked there for years. I needed to go back to the roots of what had worked for me before, and what I trusted would make a straight line of impact. I was embarrassed I didn't think of this before. Anyway, I shared with Corey my frustration and sense of defeat. He gently reminded me that four months wasn't that long and offered to help me. We did a QEEG brain scan and started a treatment program in neurofeedback, which made a huge difference. I soon felt less obsessive and more flexible, so I didn't spend as much time over-focusing on this recovery, could shift mental gears more easily, and my speech became reliable. My confidence slowly came back.

In the end, being able to think more clearly was worth the three-hour-round-trip commute to his office. My appointments were usually on Fridays and getting to geek out and listen to NPR's Science Friday while in my car was a bonus.

I am grateful I had the neurofeedback option and to work with Corey. Although even now, a year and a half later, I still feel like I am working to get back to my full peak. The lesson here is to realize you may need to pull in different tools over time.

Because a concussion and post-concussion symptoms may appear in the different domains Stoler and Hill outlined, your best strategy for a full recovery will likely be multi-dimensional. Neurofeedback is increasingly used in the rehabilitation of former professional football players. The Interactive Metronome is also a research-based tool that has been shown to improve deficits in those who have suffered a concussion, including getting executive functions (planning, decision-making, focus) online. It also helps memory, speed of information processing, and motor coordination. I used many tools in my recovery and continue to do so. Most people who work in my field have many tools they enjoy trying and using daily, not just to address injury but to help with stress and making the most out of life.

My Work Today

The focus of my private practice has not been on using applied neuroscience for treating recent concussions. I use neurofeedback for clients with issues such as peak performance, focus, depression, or anxiety. Often my clients are already peak performers who can't quite get where they want to go in their sport, work, and personal lives. Most typically, clients I see are executives, professionals, or anyone else who wants to optimize their brain to do and feel better.

Curiously, from doing brain scans, I often see clients who may have had a head injury in the past that they don't remember, like falling off a swing as a kid or bumping their head on a cabinet door in their kitchen at home. However, the imprint on their brain wave patterns is evident, even years later. Improving early forgotten injuries increases brain power and improves mood and energy.

Overall, I have worked with hundreds of people whose issues are both common and unique. I'll share some of these in the next chapter with a collection of composite cases. They illustrate how neurofeedback and an array of applied neuroscience and alternative medicine tools can help reach a range of career and life goals.

Chapter 17:

Rewired: Stories of Crisis, Challenge, and Applied Neuroscience

The more we know about brain-based tools and related health factors, the more we can help our brain in optimal ways. We can feel and function better than we ever would have otherwise as we come up against the challenges of life, including traumatic events and even aging.

This chapter will share stories about how taking an applied neuroscience approach to optimize the brain can make a life-changing difference. You will see how the tools and concepts we have been talking about extend to other issues and situations. To protect my clients' privacy, these stories are composites with all personally identifying information changed.

To summarize, my background has been in counseling and career and executive coaching. My master's degree is in clinical and counseling psychology with additional graduate-level coursework toward a doctorate in organizational psychology. I am a licensed clinical professional counselor with training in coaching and leadership development. After my accident in October 2005 and about two years of treatment and another two years of professional training, I earned a board certification in neurofeedback in 2010.

Since recovering from a traumatic brain injury in about 2008, I have been a complete learning machine. I know firsthand, life is precious and not guaranteed.

The first years of practice in what I call my "new field" using applied neuroscience tools were, therefore, somewhat different from the work I did before my accident. My internships, especially the time with Dr. Abbott, involved a clinical caseload using neurofeedback for medical concerns of depression, anxiety, and ADHD. This was different from the typical concern I hear as a coach, which was, "How can I do better at work when I hate my boss?"

Little by little in the last ten years, I have moved back to my roots focusing on peak performance for nonclinical clients because I truly believe everyone can benefit from brain science in daily life. There doesn't need to be a clinical concern at the basis and, truth be told, the issues of anxiety, depression, and focus often weave in varying degrees through "normal" people's lives. Through my recovery, I was trained in biofeedback heart rate variability training (HRV), EMDR, and as I worked longer in applied neuroscience, I wanted even more brain or physiologically based tools for my other clients. I read a great deal and completed a certification in integrated medicine and nutrition for mental health with Dr. Lesley Korn. As you may recall from earlier chapters, food science is a passion of mine, as is studying supplements and other alternative medicine practices that help the brain—yoga, meditation.

A couple more points of clarification before we go further: Some of my clients also see a psychotherapist. In that capacity, I am a specialist on the treatment team, often informally referred to as the "brain person." Being invited to this team arrangement is common for professionals who specialize and are board certified in neurofeedback. For most of my clients, I do both roles. That is, I am also their coach or psychotherapist and bring in brain-based tools as appropriate for their goals. I am hired by individuals but also organizations to help leaders and other staff. Increasingly you find more coaches and therapists are drawing upon neuroscience. I think that's a good thing.

On with our stories.

The Sad Dad: Resistant Depression

Early in the new practice, I had a client in his late thirties who I'll call Ken. He suffered from severe depression. The therapist who referred him said it was quite serious, so I consulted Dr. Abbott. We collaborated on the training protocol, then Ken and I did neurofeedback training. He had also been seeing another therapist for in-depth psychotherapy for the last five years. He started with her shortly after his father died when he slumped into a depression. Their progress was slow. Recently, he seemed to be losing some of his precious gains and, instead, was spiraling down. Ken, his therapist, and his wife all agreed he needed something. "The brain stuff" was worth a try.

Ken had a wife, Bev, and a fourteen-month-old daughter, Bella. Both Ken and Bev worked outside the home. As time passed, the weight of Ken not being a partner in raising their very active baby was weighing heavily. Ken was not present in his marriage or life. The one glimmer of humor he shared at our first meeting was describing his baby as Boisterous Bella, noting she had "the lungs of an opera singer." Behind his smile, I felt a sense of frustration and shame for his perceived inadequacy.

Ken described his workdays as dragging himself along, checking the clock, pulling himself through minute by minute, waiting for the relief of being able to leave and go home. Once he got home, all he wanted to do was sit and tune out. It's easy to imagine Ken sprawled out with feet up in his big, brown leather recliner, TV on, wearing his T-shirt and shorts, regardless of the season. Ken said after work, he wasn't just tired; he was "completely exhausted." The most energetic part of him was an incessantly self-critical voice trapped in his head constantly pelting him:

- What kind of man are you if you sit here every night in front of the TV?
- What would your father say about you if he were alive right now?
- You're a failure on every single front.
- How long do you think it will be before your wife leaves and takes your daughter?

- What good is your life, anyway?
- Would your wife and daughter be better off without you?

Each evening Ken felt more defeated and isolated. Bev was worried, and to be honest, as much as she loved him, was getting fed up. She had a husband who was either very sick or had changed a lot from the man she married. He had tried several different depression medications. Nothing made a sustained difference. Most painful, Ken was someone who she couldn't reach anymore. Finally, Bev convinced Ken to start neurofeedback and go in for an annual checkup with his physician. It had been years past due. She set up appointments for him, and he kept them.

His QEEG brain map showed the classic imprint of depression. The region of the brain that is wired for pleasure, our endogenous reward system on the left frontal lobe, had too much alpha wave activity. That dampens our ability to feel pleasure in life. The alpha pattern was asymmetric, meaning there was more slower wave activity on the left frontal lobe than the right. The left frontal lobe has to do with motivation and "approach" behavior, and with all that alpha, he was more apt to withdraw or "avoid."

Ken seemed distracted and lethargic, afraid to hope for a better life, and it was hard to add two sessions a week to his exhausting schedule. His neurofeedback treatment was an uphill climb, but he made progress.

Depression is typically the product of multiple factors, including heredity, psychology, body physiology, diet and exercise, brain activity, and environment. Ken got the results of the blood work; it showed he had a deficiency in vitamin D3. One of the possible correlates of D3 deficiency is depression. That day, Ken began taking a therapeutic dose and, across time, built up his D3 levels. We attacked depression from many angles, beginning with neurofeedback training to support brain improvement and encouraging small steps toward new health habits, such as walking, drinking more water, writing gratitude lists, and cutting sugar (which causes many people to experience mood issues).

With more energy and spirit, he was then able to dig deeper with his therapist. He had more emotional and physical stability to explore what it meant to become a father, especially as Bella was growing into a real person. His father was a man he had deeply loved, resented, and feared all at the same time.

In time, Ken found a new plane of functioning for his life. The veil of sadness, lethargy, hopelessness, and lack of pleasure lifted. He smiled more. Looking back, he can hardly believe how difficult his life had become and how close he had been to the edge of ending it. Little Bella welcomed a father who became curious about her reactions to life and delighted in making her smile. He began to act like a real team member with Bev for Bella's care. Ken and Bev looked forward to a new addition to their weekly schedule—date night on Thursdays—to snuggle up together at the movies or hold hands over dinner at their favorite restaurant while Bella entertained her grandmother.

Ken's life had changed for the better, and it impacted many. It was not surprising that when we redid his brain scan after twenty-five sessions, the areas of dysregulation had become smaller and overall looked more normal. We did another five sessions of brain training to increase his concentration power at work and then said, "goodbye for now." I'm here if he ever needs a tune-up.

Sleepless (and Anxious) in Chicago

During our initial meeting, Raj dodged eye contact by looking down a lot. Still, in small and deliberate quips, he confessed he was worried about his job, as well as his relationship with his wife. A young man in his late twenties, Raj worked as a business analyst and bore a resemblance to Harry Potter with dark hair and roundish glasses. He was worried that he didn't know what to talk about with his wife, Naila, in the morning and after getting home from work. He was also afraid she would realize he couldn't keep track of what she was saying, especially if she went on too long. Yes, sometimes his mind would just be distracted and space out. Coming back to focus on her, it felt like he was just watching her mouth move. This didn't happen just with his wife, whom he loved. This was a secret he had kept since high school or maybe even before. He would tune out in conversations, and then when he returned his attention, he didn't have a sense of what was going on. It was a lonely secret, one he never shared with anyone.

On the job, sitting at his stacked desk, the whole office left earlier than he did and they didn't look nearly as stressed as he felt. Raj shuffled out later with his leather backpack full of work to do after his wife went to sleep. His sleep was erratic and broken. Often, he stayed up too late because he couldn't easily drift off. The catalyst for making an appointment was that his evenings were soon going to be pinched; in six months, his wife Naila was having a baby. He was very worried about this house of cards all coming down at once.

One of the different types of ADHD (Attention Deficit Hyperactivity Disorder) is Inattentive Attention Deficit (often called ADD). It's the classic pattern of a person being challenged by maintaining a focus. These daydreamers may not be identified in schools or work situations as easily as someone with attention deficit with hyperactivity. With hyperactivity, you see impulsiveness, lots of fidgeting, moving around. The movement is a way of keeping the brain awake and alert. With the Inattentive ADHD, symptoms include forgetfulness, lack of focus, being easily distracted, making careless mistakes, and not following through. It can appear these people are not listening when others are talking. In Raj's case, that was often true.

Our conversations were challenging for Raj from the beginning. Later, when I knew him better, he said the "checking in" part of the session, before the neurofeedback training part, was the hardest part of the whole treatment. He didn't know what to say to me either, and his default pattern of looking intelligent and trying to listen to the other person didn't work with me. In our relationship, talking was his job, so I could know where to target the neurofeedback and how it was working.

At work, people likely saw him as an intelligent, soft-spoken, and reserved person who thought before he spoke and worked hard. Raj was all those things and more—including terrified.

Session by session, step by step, with lots of encouragement, he engaged in his treatment. It's important to appreciate the amount of courage it takes for people to reach out and risk exposing themselves to address patterns like this. In his treatment, Raj developed a voice and sense of self he didn't have before or had been dormant inside him. I am honored to be entrusted with vulnerabilities such as these.

His QEEG brain scan showed a deficit of slow waves (theta, alpha) in his occipital lobe, located in the back of the head. He could not let himself sleep completely because he was continually worried. So, we did a training called Alpha Theta to help him fall asleep, stay asleep, and sleep more deeply. The goal was to reduce the anxiety that fragmented his attention.

He would come into the office during his lunchtime, recline in a chair with his eyes closed, and put on headphones that played the sounds of rain falling and ocean waves. He learned to increase his theta waves to relax more deeply. The sounds changed to reward him for increases in alpha and theta. He joked with me (humor was a sign of progress) that he was so tired from accumulated sleeplessness that he would just pay me to let him sleep there for an hour. I assured him that relaxing deeply was the task, so no worries.

Over a series of sessions twice a week, he stopped feeling like he needed the alpha theta training and was resting well at home. Little by little, he looked more like a person who was tracking the conversation and began engaging with me. He looked more present, had opinions, and even a sense of humor.

After we finished the alpha theta training, we worked on strengthening his capacity to pay attention. This training was different since he had his eyes open, and the stimulus was watching movies or TED talks and learning about the world around him. Not only did we "rewire" his brain for the "eyes open" world, but he was exposing himself to more interesting information he would not have had before. Anxiety makes our world small or often boring. The training principle goes like this: when his brain focuses on the movie, he is rewarded by the movie being light and loud, but if he gets distracted, the show becomes dark, and the volume is lowered. So it's hard to see and hear. Over and over, this reward pattern will serve to reinforce being focused and create positive learning.

Raj and I worked together for about a year. Overall, the change was dramatic. He looked and functioned more coherently. He was "in there," so much more present and engaged in life. He became a funny, smart, skillful, kind, and thoughtful conversationalist. His wife and new baby son enjoy him, and, equally important, Raj is enjoying them.

Mysterious June: My Turning Point

Using my clinical brain-based approach with my roots in career and executive coaching began with this case in about spring 2012. I had a contract from a large consulting firm to provide coaching services to an emerging leader with their client—a large bank. The contract entailed a rich collection of many popular behavioral style and personality tools like DiSC®, Myers Briggs Type Indicator, 16 PF for Leaders and FIRO-B, and a 360-degree assessment. I love all tests since they serve as "mirrors" to identify strengths and areas for development. Clients usually find testing reports about their management and leadership skills quite powerful. These are like doing quizzes in magazines on steroids. This coaching project featured a comprehensive and expensive collection of tools.

My coachee's name was June, a banking executive. She methodically worked through the series of long personalized test reports, one each session. Unlike over ninety percent of people receiving such data, nothing seemed surprising or even mildly disconcerting to her. She stayed cool and collected. Over time, I wasn't sure why she wanted coaching. It seemed like she was checking the boxes off a list of what someone should do who wanted to move up.

One day, I noticed I had my biofeedback device in my purse and, totally off script, asked her if I could teach her coherent breathing. We clipped the device to her ear. With practice, she could breathe rhythmically and deeply enough to melt into the calm zone. She looked like a different person—so relaxed and present—but didn't say much. I asked her to do it for five minutes each morning if she could. Two weeks after we first did this breathing exercise in session, her program ended.

For the last session, we planned a coaching project debrief. She seemed like a tough customer who was unimpressed and not getting much from the whole thing. I was ready for her feedback but still dreading that now her dissatisfaction would be fully aired. When I asked her what she got from this program, she responded immediately: "I liked the breathing practice. I do it every morning."

I was surprised and asked her to say more. "I wake up and sit on the side of my bed first thing with my eyes closed. I take about five minutes. It changes everything. My husband says it helps me too. He worries about the pressure of my job." I realized she was like a little soldier who had trained herself to not outwardly show the immense stress she was feeling. Still, her husband knew it and saw that the breathing time was helping.

After that, I began bringing these self-regulation body/brain tools into all my coaching and counseling. The gap between the coaching I did before and my "new practice" was getting smaller. I now integrate and introduce whichever biofeedback and neurofeedback tools would be most helpful to each person's goals.

The Bulldozer Executive: On Female Leadership

One of my colleagues, Trevor, from a business board I was on years ago, asked me to help his company, a mid-sized technical firm. They had an employee, a team leader and principal who was excellent at her job, getting projects done and (what every company in the world would dream of) under budget. However, bodies were left along the way—lots of them. And Bulldozer became her nickname—behind her back, of course.

Her management style was loud and explosive, and her temper was short. Her team was terrorized by her moods, which had become even more volatile since her divorce a year earlier. Shondra, a mother of three college-aged kids, now in her fifties, had grown up in this organization. Super smart, she could diagnose or anticipate a system problem before anyone else and snap out orders to fix it. However, the talent of her team, difficult to find and hire, had begun leaving little by little because of her rants. Her behavior was creating a problem for the organization.

Trevor was torn since he had known Shondra for a long time and considered her a friend. He could see she was not quite herself. Instead, she was more of all her worst traits and less of her best, the same way we all can get under great stress. Trevor had a long talk with her and said, either you make some changes, and we will provide a coach, or you'll need to leave. It wasn't the first talk they had had about her manner, but it was a final one since Trevor felt the pressure from the rest of the executive committee. You could see the angst in Trevor's eyes as he described the situation. He knew Shondra wasn't in a good place, but the cost of her behavior was increasing, and she just couldn't seem to rein in her reactiveness.

Trevor had made it clear to her that working with a coach would be her decision. Coaching clearly was one of the last things she would have considered. With a divorce she didn't see coming or want, and the kids getting on with their own lives, this company was her life, and in some ways, all she had.

She agreed to meet with me for an introduction but only if we could meet in her office. She was slightly open to our working together, especially since one of her daughters was studying neuroscience. Shondra liked the idea that her daughter was impressed and decided to try the "brain stuff."

Trevor brought me to her doorway and made introductions. She sat commandingly behind the huge cherrywood desk wearing a prim, buttoned-up flowered blouse, with long painted nails, and a knee-length black pencil skirt. Behind her thick glasses and dark curly hair, her eyes betrayed her, and she looked like she was going to cry. In that instant, I knew I liked her a lot, and we would be great partners to work on her goals. She was proud and vulnerable at the same time.

She just wanted to be okay but needed help. It would not be easy for her to ask for or accept help but... I know what all that's like myself.

For me, neurofeedback is a tool and part of an integrative process. Intense stress dysregulates your brain. If your brain is dysregulated, it directly affects your emotional state. As a tool, neurofeedback makes behavioral change easier since it helps you gain control over your emotional reactions.

We never tried to zap away the pain of loss and stress in Shondra's life. I listened, she talked, tears were shed, and insights revealed themselves about how her life had evolved and what did or did not support her. She wrote in a journal between sessions, giving herself space to deal with the grief she felt over her marriage and her resentments about the company. We discussed triggers in the office for her outbursts and unprofessional behavior, as well as the vision of what she wanted for her leadership and her life. The neurofeedback training made it easier for her to tap into the feelings buried beneath her anger, get control of her actions, and generate positive as well as negative feelings. How?

To start, her brain scan was, of course, not good. It was highly dysregulated from years of stress and burnout of a hard-driving career where self-care, like her marriage, always took a back seat. Many women have trouble with self-care when others need them. We all need support to change these habits. The underpinning of her neglect explained where her energy was going, instead. The map showed her temporal lobes were "on fire" or highly active, reflecting unregulated limbic system areas. The limbic system deals with emotions, memory, and arousal. This spilled into the occipital lobe, which is concerned with sleep and anxiety. It was overactivated. That's like having your foot stuck on the gas pedal and being unable to downshift when needed. Ideas churned in her head constantly when she needed to be sleeping or at least giving herself a break. All this reduced the power in the frontal lobes, which are our brain's manager CEO. This left her victim to her basic emotional impulses at times.

Shondra gave her life willingly to her job, and now they would threaten her with termination? This is one of the many resentments this tired and overworked manager had. Anxiety distorts our awareness of our behavior; we have all been there, too. Many of her resentments were well-founded at how the good old boys treated her as a woman and a minority and how indirect and political their communications often seemed. We worked on constructive skills for dealing with this and owning her authentic power in these situations. "No need to raise your voice. You are already powerful."

She was open to the neuroscience tools and wrote her daughter notes regularly about what she was doing in our work—complete with photos she had me take on her iPhone. She trained twice a week in my downtown office largely with heart rate variability (HRV) or coherent breathing, as well as QEEG map-based neurofeedback. We first targeted sleep for her anxiety and emotional reactivity, then moved on to her QEEG imprint of depression. All this gave her more energy, resilience, and mental flexibility. Working on her brain waves in this way resulted in her seeing a situation from different angles more easily. She'd get less worked up over events that happened and switch to another priority. It all drained her less, and she had more time to live a new life she was making.

Relationships were a target area for improvement, so we strategized on some behavioral shifts in patterns with her staff. This is what I mean by process; I had learned from staff interviews that people felt she was unfriendly, and they constantly felt on guard around her. So, her assignments included practicing small new behaviors like smiling at people she was passing in the hall. Research shows that smiling releases the feel-good neurotransmitters in the brain and reduces cortisol which helps our own mood and others.

A gratitude journal was used to help restructure her thinking. Then, with the coaching nudge, an assignment was to have her tell people some of these things she was noting.

"If you are grateful your boss gave you this coaching option, what would happen if you told him that?"

These were little and big assignments to help her better shape relationships and signal that she was changing. These actions cascaded and multiplied as people reacted more positively to Shondra. She started to receive some of the social connection she longed to have. There were ups and downs and no shortage of moments in our conversations when she felt frustrated at her lack of progress (sound familiar?). Overall, Shondra made some significant changes in her behavior and her life.

This work is an honor. Architects build structures, beautiful ones. In coaching with brain-based power tools, I believe we help people build themselves and their future. I worked with Shondra for one year. In the end, her company felt she had made some significant changes, and our program ended. At about the sixth month, Shondra reflected on her behavior in the year that followed her divorce. I told her: "No worries. We all go through weird times. I certainly know that." As I write this, I hope I am never asked to coach at a company that wears green shirts. She also credits her journey for forcing her to do what she needed to do long ago—focus on self-care—but feels she's now becoming the role model she wants for her daughters.

She is more comfortable with herself and is creating a life she truly likes. Believe it or not, she took up bowling and was in a recent ad on Match.com. Her outbursts are now almost nonexistent. However, if you are working with her, not listening and should be, and a project is getting off track, rest assured that she will tell you that very directly. That doesn't always fit nicely with her male colleagues who still may call that bulldozing. However, I suspect they need coaching, too, to become more direct in their own communications.

She's great about keeping in touch. The last time she emailed, she told me that she was teaching her staff meditative breathing to "calm and center" before their group meetings. I so love my work.

One of a Kind

In many companies, either family-owned and operated, or with very specialized talent, one person can make a huge difference, whether we are talking about the president or a code-maker, manager, or other technician. If this person isn't functioning at the level needed, or can't step up to the next challenges, the company's future will bear the impact. I was contacted by a small high-profile manufacturing firm with a key high-potential member of their quality team we will call Sam. A lovable member of the team and very smart, but his ADD got the best of him. Mathematically gifted, he could make and adapt computer systems to keep up with the robots manufacturing the parts, putting in the specifications to create their products. It was stunning, but his ADD made his and everyone's life challenging at points.

An earnest man in his forties, he'd put in long hours to meet deadlines for clients. He would do whatever it took when the chips were down. But day in and day out, he had so many different projects he was working on and things half-finished that it seemed like nothing got done, despite all his hard work. He'd love to laugh and share a story with people who came in and out of his lab all day. Each conversation began with a question for him and often got sidetracked. In conversation, each sentence had several forks or trees in it. Here's an example of his conversation with me:

"Well, I wanted to talk with you about how to handle my boss. I don't think he listens to me. Did you ever see the SNL skit with Tina Fey in it? That one that... Oh, never mind, my wife's mom is visiting us this week, which makes everything more stressful at home. My kids aren't doing their homework. When I was in fifth grade, we didn't even have homework. Not like this."

Even I, a potential tree-maker myself, can get lost in his communications. Sam had issues that kept him from moving up in the organization: constant movement or fidgeting, low confidence, and challenges with speech fluency. Believe it or not, despite loving to talk, he was shy and unsure of himself in dealing with superiors. Also, his words didn't always flow naturally. He would try to articulate an idea, but it didn't always come out as smoothly as he liked, which frustrated him. Often, he laughed it off, but it undermined his confidence, and he would ruminate for hours later, reviewing his "mistakes."

The brain map showed classic ADHD attention deficit disorder with hyperactivity. We began with HRV training once a week for six months. Because my office was far away, the company arranged for Sam to have a device to use at work on break and at home. He was also to teach his teenagers, since the more a family knows about what a patient is doing, the more they can support him and benefit from it themselves.

This was an important project, and, on a whim, I decided to videotape our interviews at strategic points along the way:

- At the beginning, during goal setting
- During the QEEG testing wearing the cap that collects brain waves at 20 scalp locations simultaneously. Most clients like to have their picture taken with that on to show friends
- At the mid-point of the program
- At the end

Progress? Some people do not notice their progress, and, despite what I see, may not be convinced they are making changes. Or, if they see changes, will attribute them to something else. (Okay, I know we've talked about this before, but I am getting wiser here.) Before the neurofeedback training, I gave Sam some objective tests of the different types of memory (short-term, working, sequential), executive functions, and processing speed.

With Sam, even though the testing showed some gains on executive functions and memory, he still didn't think he changed. So, I was worried about how the debrief meeting would go with the company vice-president—the "what did you accomplish with this time and our financial investment" session. Then, I got an idea. We'd look at the video and put that together—the pre- and post-training—to see what he said.

Well, it was revealing, not because of the content of him saying what he gained (nothing overwhelming), but when you watched him, it was dramatic. His initial interview was more tentative, halting. His humor seemed thin and gratuitous. In the video of our last interview, he was confident, quick yet generous in his exchanges with me, explaining things he thought I needed more information on. He had fewer body movements and gestures, and they were more purposeful. He somehow appeared more solid. It was a stunning result that no one watching could deny.

Change is strange since we know ourselves and others in the moment, and that seems right until we can contrast it to a piece of "what was." Here is a more recent case since we took on the Interactive Metronome just over a year ago.

The Ruminator and the IM

This is a brief story of a treatment that was also brief. My assistant, Tricia, and I had the opportunity to work with a rather high-functioning consultant, Gwen. She's a bouncy, outgoing executive in her mid-forties from the field of fundraising who looks like she played competitive sports in college—strong and confident with lots of charisma.

Gwen works in a competitive field marked by intense periods of activity. During these periods, she manages and coordinates activities to create large events for clients. This entails listening carefully to understand her client's vision with all the rich nuances, problem-solving their needs and budgets, meeting unexpected demands from high-profile donors, interfacing with vendors of all kinds, meeting many new people at once, remembering a sea of names, and staying focused and calm. As Gwen has grown older, she's become more and more concerned about staying at the top of her game since, for example, forgetting a major donor's name can have high stakes. Her goals for our program were to strengthen memory and to increase productive focus by wasting less time on rumination and second-guessing.

Anxiety is often at the core of how people waste energy. Passive and anxious people get stuck, demotivated, and can occasionally say hateful things to themselves. Action-oriented anxious people often use their busy brain against themselves by lying awake ruminating and second-guessing their activities.

The project was structured by the client's desire to do the Interactive Metronome (IM), the behaviorally based brain training (aka "clapping and slapping"). Gwen came in twice a week for six weeks total, with a break of a week in the middle, and worked with Tricia and/or me doing the IM exercises. In total, she did twelve sessions of about fifty minutes each.

The movement exercises are work because most of us don't use our upper bodies even for clapping to a rhythm in short segments. But Gwen was hardy, wore her gym clothes, peeling off layers when she started to perspire, and overall, personally showed up. She loved the biohacking element of knowing that the research showed she could, and would, make a difference to her brain. This training is not watching a TED Talk or listening to tinkly sounds with earphones on your head. This is for the hardy, and many of our clients, especially athletes, feel great for having done this unique workout. Like most, she did get pinkish looking as we challenged her outside limits by increasing the number of repetitions she did for different parts of the body. But Gwen said she felt like she was waking up her body as well as her brain.

She started to notice differences within three or four sessions. One example she gave was hearing a phone number a client rattled off on a call. Now she was more likely to think she could remember it long enough to write it down versus feeling panicked. She was finding it easier to make task lists and check them off. Things felt clearer, and this made decisions—and there are many in her work—come a lot faster. She was more willing to decide and put her stake in the ground to defend things, if needed. It was a relief to find more objectivity. While we never promised better sleep from the IM, as time went on and things felt less murky (strengthening the executive functions), she did sleep better. She could "rest assured."

At the end of twelve sessions, or six training weeks, Gwen was quite happy with her outcomes. Our benchmark testing showed many gains in our target areas of attention, focus, rumination, second-guessing, and task productivity. Since it was early in the year, we didn't get to find out how one last detail went. Tricia and I were hoping, as we saw in the IM research literature, that Gwen's golf game would show some gains too. Here's hoping she had some great games of golf after her training success.

It's easy to underestimate how valuable it is to increase people's confidence in how their brain works. It reduces stress to have better cognitive skills. I mentioned I used the IM after my second concussion. I still go back and *occasionally* do some of the exercises for a workout. My memory is especially good, not perfect, but good. Because it wasn't good after the recent concussion, I feel as though I created this result and am happy with that. To use a popular term—biohacked!

Many Stories—Athletes, Migraines, Career Fog, and Physician Burnout

I could tell you stories forever from my own experiences, from those of my clients as well as from clients of my colleagues. Other favorites include mitigating the maddening migraines of mothers and lawyers, tackling Tourette's tics, accessing and creating emotional resources for assault victims, and easing the withdrawal of one of the many people I have seen who were prescribed benzodiazepines before anyone realized what a hell-pit the withdrawal can be. Two areas especially important to me lately are:

Career and Stress

As a career coach, over the years, I noticed that prolonged stress from a poor job fit or work environment can make it very challenging, even impossible, for people to figure out who they are and what they want. Now in working with these types of clients, I often suggest some level of neuroscience-based support and self-regulation practice (e.g., meditation or breathing practice, neurofeedback) to help them regroup before deciding about what's best for them. If you've had a bad job that's made you wonder who you are and what to do next, or even if you have lost your job, try out some of the tools I described in my own treatment and within these above client stories. Reground yourself, connect to your intuition, and it will make you feel stronger.

Physicians and Suicide

Chicago is a town with many large hospitals, and health care is a stressful field. I have coached and done neurofeedback training with several physicians who suffer from burnout, anxiety, and depression.

Doctors are a very stressed group, and I love working with them. We think together about their patterns and challenges. Drawing from brain science and integrative medicine creates protocols on how they can best proceed. We examine what they're eating, their environments, any medications they take, and exercise. They are scientists. They get it. They need space to not be in charge and get assistance to care for themselves. It's rewarding to help them access deep restorative sleep, resilience, leadership skills, and compassion, especially for themselves.

Often physicians, especially those in training, have long, stressful hours. They routinely confront the uncompromising pulls of competing demands from corporate goals and mandates, patient needs, and insurance companies with broken systems. Often the medications and the care patients may critically need are not based on practicality. It's a high-stakes game with less time to do what brought most of them into the profession—listen to and help their patients. A sense of purpose grounds us and reduces the likelihood of burnout. Says Dr. Linda Girgis, Editor-in-Chief of *Physician's Weekly*:

"The stress on doctors has never been as much as it is today... Burnout has never been more common, and we can only expect it to continue to rise. Sadly, many doctors feel the only way out is suicide. While many people are aware of the problem of burnout, few are offering reasonable solutions. Resiliency training or mindfulness is not going to cure our burnout when the system is broken, and no one is working to fix it."

Physician suicide rate is high. Brilliant men and women are pushed to the edge. They need tools to help them cope with increasingly complex and demanding jobs and to fortify their resilience. Their strength is needed to rally for the change in the systems that are a major contributor to such unforgiving desperation.

Hopefully, this chapter provided ideas to help you and your friends and family understand how a life comes undone and how the tools of neuroscience and integrative medicine can help create new footing.

https://www.webmd.com/mental-health/news/20180508/
doctors-suicide-rate-highest-of-any-profession#1

Chapter 18:

The Self, Second Chances, Neuroscience, and the Future

Sense of Self and the Brain

People have asked me if this moderate concussion changed me, altered who I am as a person. I want to immediately say, "No. I am the same, and can do everything I could before." But that's not true. When our brain changes, we change. When we change, our brain changes. After the accident, my sense of who I was collapsed inward. Within a few months, most of my key self-identifying activities and accomplishments were diminished or had slipped away. These big things included Tae Kwon Do Club, the movement part as well as the social contact, presentations on my book that had been recently released, the Toastmaster's group I attended for two years with the great friendships developed there and, for a while, even driving my car. My brain's GPS went a little awry and instead helped build me a safe mental place deep inside where I lived with my wonderful husband. I was like a small snail, stunned and safe, who didn't move around too much.

Little by little, the presence of other people—Dr. Locke, my friend Georgia, Elsa Baehr, Dr. Kathy Abbott, Eckhart Tolle, Thich Nhat Hanh, and Judy Crawford—provided tools or support to move ahead. But it was a slow process because I wasn't only moving; I was transforming, evolving into someone different, someone with a wider view and more depth.

In each stage, I had to lose my skin to move to the next. I had to learn to live with not knowing or being able to look ahead at what would happen since all of what was me was taken or turned upside down. I was lucky to come across great teachers to help me with life, to be grateful and stay in the moment, to sit in these undefined and unexpected spaces, and eventually use them to create the next steps. I spent time with my dragons, though. It wasn't easy. We transform our lives, but our lives transform us.

On the cognitive level, especially still recovering from Pru2, my overall memory is good, but my short-term memory is not as strong as before. That means if you told me something in a conversation, there is a chance it might be gone from my brain by the end of the conversation. However, I have an astonishing recall of client case details, but the context in which I collect those details is very focused. When a client sits across from me in my office, all my attention goes toward listening to that person.

My speech can still be halting like it was after the accident, with the words in my mind not making it to my mouth. This happens especially if I am tired or under a lot of stress. Inside I struggle with it sometimes, but people like my husband and close friends tell me they don't notice an impairment. If I did the IM more regularly, I am confident it would mitigate that problem and increase speech fluency. But my self-care routine just feels too long some days, and I would much rather help my clients than myself. Don't be fooled. I take excellent care of myself overall.

Some say these speech challenges come with age. It's been fourteen years since the car accident, which brings me past sixty years old. While I don't discount the idea that the brain will change with age, I don't accept this as a limitation that I can't improve or eradicate. I just don't.

Overall, I have a better understanding of my focus and concentration issues. My concentration is impacted significantly by my diet. Having added sugar (an extremely rare event) in my diet makes my brain feel like I'm watching television with a frenetic person who's constantly clicking the remote and changing channels. To be honest, I like that feeling sometimes, and ADD suits my personality—creative, lots of ideas. I also have a little depression that never seems to completely dissipate. But I had reoccurring bouts of depression before the accident. They are triggered by stress, and the injury was a significant stressor.

On the other hand, as a close friend pointed out, I have had huge gains from this event in terms of skill development, personality, and life wisdom—all gifts of my concussions. Here are some of these gifts along with insights and recommendations I have if you had an injury or even if you haven't.

You May Be More than You Know

Having an injury can scrape your skin off, but it doesn't mean you won't or can't grow. Injuries can also help take the blinders off and bring you to another place where maybe you are meant to be. I now have things I would have never dreamed of in my pre-accident life. My professional practice is a huge example. I also have deeper relationships with people I know and love and can be truthful with them. I have more mentors than anyone deserves. I am kinder and more patient with myself and others.

My story is about more than injury, suffering, and loss. Yes, it was that—all of that and more. I am now more than I ever imagined I would be. You, too, are probably way more than you ever thought you would be. Even if life has left you cognitively and/or physically disabled and unable to leave your home, we live in amazing times, and the world is at your computer. Explore, spread your wings, see what calls you.

Trust Your Intuition

At the many points on my path to recovery, I took what felt like crazy random turns that intuition orchestrated. These became stones beneath the water, creating a path forward over what would have been otherwise impossible. Finding the church that had been at the end of our block for more than fifteen years, talking with Georgia, finding Elsa, and experiencing my retreat with Thich Nhat Hanh all had much deeper meaning than I was able to absorb at the time. Our brain shifts, we shift and find new paths, the brain seems to create new healing pathways.

I encourage you to trust, to stay open to randomness. We must learn to trust ourselves to find our way through even the most difficult times by listening to our intuition and find the stones on the perhaps hidden path forward. No matter how lost you feel and how little you know yourself at the time, trust this.

Give Yourself Time to Travel and Bring Eckhart

I encourage you to create space in life to just be, or life it seems will create it for us. Like my trips to see Elsa. Four trains and a taxi, with headphones on listening to Eckhart Tolle, accepting what was. Be mindful of life on its own terms and breathe into life. Exhale out your confusion and distrust; inhale a sense of abundant possibilities. Just as we cannot judge ourselves harshly and still grow, we cannot judge others and grow either. Let go of judgment. Be a good traveler.

Compassion Reset

Even fourteen years later, one of the biggest changes in my life remains a deeper sense of compassion and connection I feel for others, especially if they are injured. We are all vulnerable—all of us. No one is above the effects of the kinds of chance events that could happen in an instant without our permission or knowledge. Every day that I live with a well-functioning brain and am able-bodied, I am immensely grateful. I also learned a lot about the humanity of those of us who have cognitive or physical challenges. We are all in this together by different strokes of luck, learning what we can. Nothing is to be taken for granted. Love what is.

A Belief in Second Chances

Many people with injuries like mine and much worse don't find treatment or people to help them pull their lives together to begin anew. They have an accident, and things are never quite the same or certainly not better. I was given consideration and care by others outside my own circles to develop new confidence and skills, to learn to trust myself again, and to create the life my family and I can be proud of. I live each day in appreciation for the opportunities provided by Elsa Baehr and all the others who helped me recover and thrive. I owe it to them to help others who need a second chance too and encourage you to do the same.

I learned that everyone deserves a second chance at creating a life that brings satisfaction and helps the world. If you find yourself judging someone because they are poor, homeless, in prison or have been, or not performing well at work or being a parent, don't judge. Keep in mind the brain is a powerful factor, and they may not have had the opportunity or resources to care for their brain or to develop that you have had. Give others and yourself an opportunity for change— you can change, they can change, we all can change.

Related to this, support brain health as a human right that we are all entitled to have—giving children and adults an opportunity for healthy food, time to breathe or meditate.

Mindfulness—Using the Brain to Not Think

We must continue to learn more about the brain and to realize that how we feel in the moment is neither "the truth" or prophecy. It's how we feel in that moment. But thoughts and feelings are changeable. Higher thinking can intervene if we cultivate it. Through meditation, neurofeedback, prayer, connection with our environment and our tribe, we can come out in a better place. More generosity, equanimity, and compassion can prevail. With practice, these brain shifts can happen much faster. That's where science needs to be—finding how we can bring our best brain and heart to the world and each other.

Mindfulness, even when I was a protective little snail, saved me. At so many moments, I tried to practice staying out of my head and in my body, feeling whatever feelings occurred. Finding the stillness and peace beneath whatever else is pulling our attention helps heal us.

Love Heals? Well... Not Quite

Love does make a difference in healing and helping us be the best we can be. But when I learn about a new neurofeedback protocol from my case group to treat my migraine client, and it reduces her headaches from four times a week to once a month, that's science. And that science means there will be fifteen days fewer a month when her little boy comes home from school to a mom who is not thick with medications, zoned out on the couch feeling morally and physically defeated by an illness that defies her control. Instead, she can be emotionally available for her precious one, be his mom, the one she always wanted to be, and the one he needs. Every parent and child deserve these opportunities. When after twelve sessions of applied neuroscience training, my burnt-out executive begins to restore her sense of personal dignity by becoming more emotionally centered, better able to collaborate with difficult people, and more effective at managing her subordinates with calm and compassionate decision-making, science is there too. Science, especially neuroscience, can help our world.

Love isn't enough. That is, unless you're talking about the love of my teachers and other scientists and practitioners who move our field of applied neuroscience forward. These are people like Elsa Baehr, Kathy Abbott, the Thompsons, Tom Collura, and Richard Soutar, who have devoted long hours to teaching, learning, and working with our dynamic technologies. Many people may not know much about these professionals and may not even consider their services because of health insurance coverage deficits. Still others may want a quicker solution, preferably one that can be taken easily with a glass of water. Understandable.

Yet increasingly, in this awesome period of breakthroughs in technology and neuroscience, life is leading us down another path, toward the magic of ways to manage the brain through applied neuroscience. My hope is that this path will lead us all to a more enduring, healthier, and fulfilling life. Thank you for sharing my journey so far.

Acknowledgements

Bringing *Brain Dance* to fruition involved a collection of people and groups without whom, the book would not have happened. As the project took shape, my life continued to change, heal, and grow creating an unbelievable network of people. This section is to acknowledge those not already mentioned in the body of the book and there are many.

But first, my husband Gary, a journalist himself, experienced my whole concussion journey and helped make sense of it. He was always there to listen and help sort our lives. We laughed and cried through the writing process and he was there any time I needed a quick review of an early draft. His spirit is generous and If you have read Brain Dance, you know there aren't enough words to describe Gary's extraordinary character and partnership in my life.

Katherine Foran, my friend, former neighbor, and book midwife also had important input on my first book in 2004. We had lost touch after my car accident and she never understood why until I asked if she could take a look at an early draft of *Brain Dance*. The more I wrote, she read, and we talked, the more we both understood how the story of my injury was, in fact, a part of our friendship story. Nothing difficult had happened between us, I had just gone into my shell. That calcified and limited my life in ways that needed to change to write this book and reclaim parts of my life. Renewing and deepening our relationship during this process has been an unexpected gift.

As an editor and journalist, K (as she goes by) has many strengths. She's brilliant and can ask difficult questions and give feedback in ways you can hear. She reviewed several drafts and helped anchor the project with her resolute belief that I had a story to share, that I was worthy of sharing it and that could I write this. Grateful for her help in doing that.

When I presented my book idea at the Harvard Medical School Writing, Publishing and Social Media for Healthcare Professionals conference in June 2019, as described in the Introduction, I had just begun to write. Feeling affirmed from the experience, my goal was to finish the manuscript by the next conference in 2020 in hopes of finding a publisher there.

During the year between, I was so grateful for the support of many writers I had met at that conference – some of whom have become invaluable friends. I felt a kinship among people I met at "Harvard Writers," even with those who attended the program in years previous. Many keep in touch on social media supporting each other's work – some at a distance and some more consistently. Celebrating the birth of a book is always joyous. These wonderful and inspiring people include Linda Girgis, M.D, Julie Silver, M.D, Zinaria Williams, M.D., Dr. Lisa Deguire, Jill Grimes, M.D., Sarah Gray, PsyD., Kevin Barhydt, Saul Rosenthal, PhD. Lynelle Schneeberg, PsyD, Carmen Greene, M.D, Kristin Semmelmeyer, PsyD., Joel Salinas, M.D, Susan White, DO. and James Zender, PhD.

Committed to finishing *Brain Dance* within a year, I also began working with Sara Connell in her Thought Leadership Academy (TLA). Sara is an exceptional writing coach who leads this program. Its focus is on connecting deeply with the mission of our work and living that alignment, this was perfect for me. Through TLA, I had the great benefit of Katie Kizer and Mary Balice Nelligan who provided editorial support. TLA provides a collaborative environment where "students" often help each other in little and big ways. I am especially grateful to Toby Dorr, Melanie Weller, Sherry Frey, Robin Pollak, Amy S. Peele and Josh Friedberg.

I was close to my goal of having a completed manuscript for the annual Harvard conference in April 2020 and then came the Covid-19 pandemic which put the brakes on finding a publisher. Then, in late August a dear family friend who had always been interested in my work provided an unsolicited and generous fund to have *Brain Dance* published. It was an unbelievable nudge to finish the book by taking away any of the practical barriers. "The world needs inspiring stories at this time, and I want you to be able to share yours," my friend Barcy (Barbara) Grauer said. Her friendship over 30 years and being a part of her beautiful life, has been the best gifts of all. I thank her for helping me with this dream.

At my publisher MindStir Media, I am grateful for Project Manager Jen McNabney, Paula Wiseman, editor extraordinaire and the inspiring MindStir Media founder, J.J. Hebert.

Thanks to early draft readers including Corey Feinberg, Martin Gremlich, Georgia Andrianopolos, PhD, Megan Buckley, PhD and Deborah Stokes, PhD. Megan had worked for a New York City literary agency for my first book. From Ireland, where she now lives, spent some time with my manuscript and enthusiastically affirmed the story needed to be shared.

My thanks to the advance readers, dear friends and colleagues, who have been on my journey to some degree and all of whom reviewed the manuscript just prior to publication for subject matter and readability issues: Jim Dwyer, MD, Amy Edgar, APRN, Leah Lagos, PsyD, Inna Khazan, PhD, Kathy Abbott, Psy. D., Linda Girgis, MD, Maddie Girardi, PT, Sara Connell, Sarah Gray, Psy.D., Saul Rosenthal, PhD, Richard Soutar, PhD, June Tanoue, MPH, Roshi Robert Joshin Althouse, Jill Grimes, MD, Melanie Weller, PT, Toby Dorr, Joanne Telser-Frère, DTM, James F. Zender, PhD, Laura Wimbish-Vanderbeck, PhD, Julia Eckersley, MD, Erik Messamore, MD, Dr. Celeste Grimard and Reverend Alan Taylor.

Melanie Weller pointed me to the cover art for *Brain Dance* and insisted that I give it a look. I'm grateful to artist Duy Huynh of Lark and Key for sharing his beautiful work on the cover. His wife, artist Sandy Snead, helped create the cover layout as did Dan Schiffmacher and Mindstir Media.

I'm fortunate to have long-time artist friends who grace my life with a wealth of inspiration especially Michelle Wrighte, Christine

Steyer, Paul Geiger, Ann Latinovich, Juliana Engles Storms, Peter Storms, Anne Garcia-Romero and Curt Powell. Their presence and friendship mean the world to me.

Artist Ann Latinovich provided my photo for the book jacket.

Special thanks to my assistant, the kind and brilliant Cameron Wyant, who keeps me on track. She has contributed in countless ways to balance my professional work and the writing and sharing Brain Dance.

I am so grateful for clients with whom I am entrusted their own dreams and concerns. Being a coach, therapist and applied neuroscientist is the greatest honor I can imagine. Also grateful for friends and organizations who support my practice while we support theirs including EEGChicago.com, AAPB's Michelle Cunningham and NewMind Maps' – Jordyn Judge and Shawn Bearden.

I have huge appreciation for the people and tribes not yet mentioned yet who helped me stay sane, productive, and inspired including Laura Wimbish-Vanderbeck, Maddie Gerardi, Gordon Brumwell, Ben Tanzer, the Buddhist Group within Unity Temple, Terry Kinzie, Lisa and Bruce Files, my siblings especially sister Sharon Calkins, brothers Tom and Dan Grimard and niece, Janice Gervais.

Lastly, *Brain Dance* allows me to shine a light on the life and work of Dr. Elsa Baehr. She is more than a special person in just my recovery, Elsa has positively impacted many lives. A brilliant scientist, clinician, and human with a great heart, it should be recognized that she is actually a pioneer in the field of neurofeedback. Female scientists can be overlooked in history, neither seen nor celebrated. Brain Dance is privileged to honor her.

Notes

Chapter 1: In an Instant

1. John P. Cunha. "What Facts Should I Know About Concussion." 2019.
   https://www.emedicinehealth.com/concussion/article_em.htm
   (accessed on July 6, 2020).

2. International Concussion Society. "Concussion Myths Debunked." https://www.concussion.org/news/concussion-myths-debunked/ (accessed on July 6, 2020).

3. Jeanne Marie Laskus. *Concussion*. (New York, NY: Random House, 2015).

4. Centers for Disease Control and Prevention. "What is a Concussion?" February 12, 2019.
   https://www.cdc.gov/headsup/basics/concission_whatis.html.
   (accessed on July 6, 2020).

Chapter 3: That Undefined Space

5. Jill Bolte Taylor. *My Stroke of Insight: A Brain Scientist's Personal Journey*. (Detroit: Large Print Press, 2008).

Chapter 5: What I Could Not See

6. Elsa Baehr, Peter Rosenfeld, Rufus Baehr. "Clinical Use of an Alpha Asymmetry Neurofeedback Protocol in the Treatment of Mood Disorders". *Journal of Neurotherapy 4*, no. 4 (2001), http://www.isnr-jnt.org/article/view/17168. (accessed on June 6, 2020).

7. Mayo Foundation for Medical Education and Research. "Post Concussion Syndrome."
   https://www.mayoclinic.org/diseases-conditions/post-concussion-syndrome/symptoms-causes/syc-20353352. (accessed on July 6, 2020).

8. Oliver Sacks. *The Man Who Mistook His Wife for a Hat: And Other Clinical Tales.* (New York, NY: Simon & Schuster, 1998).

9. Treatment Advocacy Center. "Anosognosia." https://www.treatmentadvocacycenter.org/key-issues/ anosognosia#:~:text=Anosognosia%2C%20also%20called%20 %22lack%20of,or%20do%20not%20seek%20treatment. (accessed on July 6, 2020).

10. National Alliance on Mental Illness. "Anosognosia." https://www.nami.org/About-Mental-Illness/Common-with-Mental-Illness/Anosognosia. (accessed on February 24, 2020).

Chapter 6: Levying the Costs

11. Daniel G. Amen. *Change Your Brain, Change Your Life: the Revolutionary, Scientifically Proven Program for Conquering Anxiety, Depression, Obsessiveness, Anger and Impulsiveness.* (New York: Times Books, 1998).

12. Eckhart Tolle. *Stillness Speaks.* (Novato, California: Namaste Publishing, 2003).

13. Eckhart Tolle. *The Power of Now.* (Novato, CA. New World Library, 2004).

Chapter 7: The Brain Training Begins!

14. Stephen Elliot and Dee Edmonson. *The New Science of Breath: Coherent Breathing for Autonomic Nervous System Balance, Health, and Well-being.* (Allen, Texas: Coherence Press, 2006).

15. John N. Demos. *Getting Started with Neurofeedback.* (New York: Norton & Co., 2005).

16. Leah Lagos, PsyD. *Heart Breath Mind: Train Your Heart to Conquer Stress and Achieve Success.* Houghton Mifflin Harcourt (August 11, 2020).

17. Inna Khazan, PhD, BCB, BCB-HRV. and Donald Moss, PhD, BCB, BCN, BCB-HRV. *Mindfulness, Acceptance, and Compassion in Biofeedback Practice.* The Association of Applied Psychophysiology and Biofeedback, Inc, 2020.

Chapter 9: The Power of Dreams

18. Brene Brown. "The Power of Vulnerability." TEDxHouston. 2010. https://www.youtube.com/watch?v=X4Qm9cGRub0

19. John N. Demos. *Getting Started with Neurofeedback.* (New York: Norton & Co., 2005).

20. Elsa Baehr, Peter Rosenfeld, Rufus Baehr, and Carolyn Earnest. "Comparison of Two EEG Asymmetry Indices in Depressed Patients vs. Normal Controls." *International Journal of Psychophysiology* 31, no. 1 (1998): 89-92.

Chapter 10: Second Chances

21. Unitarian Universalist Association, Congregational Covenants. "Griswold Williams Covenant of the Universalist tradition." https://www.uua.org/re/tapestry/adults/river/workshop7/175905.shtml. (accessed on January 17, 2021).

Chapter 11: Just When I Thought I Was Done!

22. Google Dictionary. "Trauma."

23. Francine Shapiro. *Eye Movement Desensitization and Reprocessing (EMDR): Basic Principles, Protocols, and Procedures,* 2nd Edition Second Edition The Guilford Press; Second edition (August 6, 2001).

Chapter 12: About That Bagel

24. Stanley Burroughs. *Master Cleanse.* (Burroughs Books, 1976).

25. J. J. Virgin. *The Virgin Diet.* (London: HarperCollinsPublishers, 2014).

26. Josh Axe. *The Gut Repair Cookbook: 101 Recipes That Will Nourish and Delight Your Gut.* Axe Wellness, LLC, 2016.

27. Leslie Korn, PhD. *The Good Mood Kitchen: Simple Recipes and Nutrition Tips for Emotional Balance.* W. W. Norton & Company; 1st edition (September 12, 2017)

Chapter 13: Learning, Learning, Learning

28. Diane Grimard Wilson. *Back in Control: How to Stay Sane, Productive and Inspired in Your Career Transition.* (Sentient Publications, 2004).

29. Dwelling Happily in the Present Moment, From Interbeing: Fourteen Guidelines for Engaged Buddhism (1998). by Thich Nhat Hanh with permission of Parallax Press, www.parallax.org.

30. Michael Thompson and Lynda Thompson. *The Neurofeedback Book.* (Association for Applied Psychophysiology and Biofeedback, 2015).

31. Anne Lamott. *Bird by Bird.* (New York: Anchor Books, 1997).

32. Jeanette Norden, PhD. *Understanding the Brain.* A DVD Series from Great Books: The Teaching Company, 2007.

Chapter 14: Board Certification Exam — Take One!

33. Biofeedback Certification International Alliance. BCIA.org.

Chapter 16: Lessons on Concussion

34. Diane Roberts Stoler and Barbara Alber Hills. *Coping with Concussion and Mild Traumatic Brain Injury: A Guide to Living with the Challenges Associated with Post Concussion Syndrome and Brain Trauma.* Avery, 2013.

35. Seth J. Ghillihan, PhD "The Healing Power of Telling Your Trauma Story." *Psychology Today*, 2019. (accessed July 6, 2020).

36. Taylor Norris. "What's The Difference Between Cod Liver Oil and Fish Oil?" *Healthline*, 2018. (accessed on July 6, 2020).

37. Alice Alexander, MD. https://uamshealth.com/category/medical-myths/page/4/ (last accessed January 17, 2021).

38. Eileen Gable, MD. Opthamologist, Loyola University Hospital System, Maywood Illinois. February, 2018.

39. Lynn Lennon, RN. Richmond Peak Performance, Richmond Virginia. July, 2018.

40. James F. Zender, PhD. *Recovering From Your Car Accident: The Complete Guide to Reclaiming Your Life*. Rowman & Littlefield Publishers (October 30, 2020).

Chapter 17: Rewired: Stories of Crisis, Challenge, and Applied Neuroscience

41. Pauline Anderson. "Doctors' Suicide Rate Highest of Any Profession". WebMD. (accessed on July 6, 2020).

Book Group Discussion Guide

Chapter 1: In an Instant
- Have you ever had a concussion? How did it impact you?
- Are there other times in your life when a single, unexpected instance changed your life trajectory?

Chapter 2: Wonder Woman... Almost
- Have you ever had so much resolve about acting or performing in a certain what that you could not evaluate your readiness to do it that clearly? You want something so much that but can't trust your judgement about if it's right for you in the moment?

Chapter 3: That Undefined Space
- Have you ever been in a situation where your mental or emotional capacities have been diminished? If so, what was the best and worst part?

Chapter 4: But I Love Your Shoes!
- Can you relate to the symptoms Diane was experiencing? Or, being out-of-sync with others because of what was going on with you or your perceptions?

Chapter 5: What I Could Not See
- Have you ever been at a big crossroads and felt really lost?
- Do you have a favorite role model? What are they like?

Chapter 6: Levying the Costs
- What's the biggest commitment you've had to make to have your life and health?

Chapter 7: The Brain Training Begins!

- Have you ever done neurofeedback brain training? If yes, what was it like? If no, would you like to try it?

Chapter 8: The Impatient Patient

- Have you ever done something you regret? Under what conditions might that behavior surface for you?

Chapter 9: The Power of Dreams

- Dreams are powerful. Do you have dreams that are guiding your life? What are these dreams?

Chapter 10: Second Chances

- Are you likely to give others a second chance? When is the last time you gave someone in trouble a second chance?
- Have you ever had an unexpected "freeze" response like I did after my testimonial? How did you understand it when it happened?

Chapter 11: Just When I Thought I Was Done!

- Have you ever known someone with PTSD or experienced it yourself?
- Have you tried EMDR? If not, would you like to do so? If yes, for what?

Chapter 12: About That Bagel

- Can you identify foods that change your mood or cognitive abilities?
- Try keeping a log for three days by writing down food (anything that goes into your mouth), your mood and exercise. Look for patterns.

Chapter 13: Learning, Learning, Learning

- What is your preferred way to learn? Is it from hearing lectures, reading books, getting your hands around things?
- Have you ever tried coloring as an adult? What was it like?

Chapter 14: Board Certification Exam—Take One!

- Have you ever had a pocket of feelings that surprised you? Feelings you didn't realize were there until a crisis triggered them? If so, what was that like?

Chapter 15: Life Continues: Milestones and Then the Unthinkable

- What tribes do you belong to currently? How adequately does your current life meet your needs for being a part of groups of kindred spirits?

Chapter 16: Lessons on Concussion

- Which of these concussion suggestions describe activities you currently do?
- Any of these that you would like to add (whether you have a concussion or not)?

Chapter 17: Rewired: Stories of Crisis, Challenge, and Applied Neuroscience

- Which of the stories in Chapter 17 do you identify with the most? And, why?

Chapter 18: The Self, Second Chances, Neuroscience, and the Future

- What speaks to you most in Chapter 18? What will you do different as a result of reading it?
- What's your biggest insight from having read this book? How will that impact your life?

Index

CPSIA information can be obtained
at www.ICGtesting.com
Printed in the USA
LVHW092209030521
686347LV00002B/273